MW00791641

LOOKING FOR JAZZ
A Memoir about the Black College and
Southern Town That Changed My Life
Anna R. Holloway

Published by Anna R. Holloway
For more information, visit:
annahollowaywrites.com
email: anna@annahollowaywrites.com

Don L Lee (Haki Madhubuti), "But He Was Cool" printed by permission
from Third World Press.
Cover photographs were provided by the Fort Valley State University
Heritage Room.

Cover designed by Kasun2050
Book design by Michael Campbell, MC Writing Services

ISBN: 979-8-9885148-0-0

PRAISE FOR
Looking for Jazz

"In this colorful and inspiring memoir, Professor Anna Holloway provides a touching and compelling account of her experiences as one of the earlier white instructors to teach at a public black land-grand college in the deep south during the late sixties and early seventies and the decades thereafter. Her heartwarming story will make you sad and happy at times as you reflect on the state of race relations in America today. This is a must read!"

LARRY EUGENE RIVERS is Distinguished Professor of History at Florida A&M University and a former president of The Fort Valley State University. He is the author or co-author of nine books, including his most recent, *Father James Page: An Enslaved Preacher's Climb to Freedom.*

"With amazingly crisp details, Anna Holloway warm-heartedly recounts her memories of being a white professor at black Fort Valley State College. Hers is a story of a dedicated English teacher, but also of a young woman from the Midwest who is immersed in the tensions of race in the deep South during the profound social shifts of the late 1960s. Readers familiar with Pat Conroy's *The Water Is Wide* will enjoy Holloway's insights into the culture of the black college, as well as her daring in claiming her own happiness."

ANTHONY GROOMS, author of *Bombingham* and *The Vain Conversation*

"Full of dialogue and stories, this memoir gives an insider's peek into the life of a young college instructor from the north, teaching in the south in the late 1960s and early '70s. It recalls the author's experiences settling into a new community different than the ones she knew, and forging through the challenges of her early adult life. Her unique journey led her on a path to raising a family and serving for 46 years at Fort Valley State University."

JOHN CHRISTOPHER FRAME, author of *Homeless at Harvard*, and *7 Attitudes of the Helping Heart*

"This story is a riveting account of a young Caucasian woman's complete immersion into the black culture of the south that lasts a lifetime. The protagonist takes the reader on a journey that begins when she is barely out of University, accepting a teaching position at a predominately black college. She quickly learns about the separation of white and black cultures, which is foreign to her experiences in northern states, and is a chilling commentary on the disparate and often negligent treatment of poor blacks in the south. Despite the differences she encounters, she is welcomed with open arms and accepted by her peers and her students. This is a story of courage, wonder, romance, and coming-of-age fulfillment."

PAUL CARR, author of the Sam Mackenzie and Michael Dalton mystery novels

"I grew up about thirty miles from Fort Valley State University (then Fort Valley State College), and Anna Holloway's personal story is one I wouldn't have missed for the world. I would have grabbed it off the shelf wanting to know what it was like for a young white English teacher from the Midwest to arrive at what was then an all-Black college in a small southern town.

The heart of this book, which begins in the turbulence of the late 1960s, turns out to be the writer herself—wide-eyed to start with—making friends and adapting to her new world with a calm grace as she gradually settles in, makes new friends and eventually even finds a new love. This story isn't just about her arrival in the smalltown South. It's about her finding her home there."

CHARLOTTE MOORE, author, Hunter Jones Mystery series

"Young white woman from a monocultural Midwestern town moves to the Deep South to teach English literature at one of America's historically black colleges: What could possibly go wrong? Anna's memoir of her journey from a 'white bread' background to becoming part of a rural black community in Georgia is wonderful. Armed with a treasure-trove of the British literature she had mastered at a top land-grant university in the North, Anna was clearly an inspirational and challenging professor whose students taught her almost as much as she taught them. With her words, she paints a vivid picture of the many observations that lead to new discoveries and insights—taking us from marriage to her high school sweetheart through the life changes that led to a maturing romance and raising a family with the handsome young African American who became the father of her children. Dr. Holloway has given us an inspirational look into what it felt like to traverse what were at the time two separate worlds in America."

LUANNA MEYER, author of *Bella's Legacy*

"Anyone old enough to read a newspaper in the 1960s remembers the turmoil and social change going on in America. Anna Holloway had a front-row seat. *Looking for Jazz* is a refresher course for all of that, plus a personal look at a young white woman's journey through those turbulent times. From the Vietnam War and anti-war protests, to interpersonal and structural racism and the Black Power movement, sexual harassment, southern culture and women's fashions, this fascinating glimpse into Holloway's life as an instructor at a black southern college, and a newly-wed soldier's wife, is a fascinating and entertaining time capsule. Holloway's distinctive characters and colorful details allow the reader to fully experience this memorable time in America."

MARGARET RODEHEAVER, author of *Hidden Treasure* and other novels and children's books

*"Looking for Jazz: A Memoir about the Black College and
Southern Town That Changed My Life,* is a wonderfully
written trip down memory lane! Having grown up in Fort
Valley, Georgia, many of the people and incidences described
were vivid reminders of stories I had been told, of the racial
politics that underscored everyday interactions, and of people
who impacted my life as a Fort Valley State student in the
early 1980s. Dr. Holloway interweaves rich details about
her journey from the lily-white Midwest to the unfamiliar
customs of a black college in central Georgia, where she
ultimately settled down and raised a family. A page-turner
from beginning to end, the imagery and rich details coalesce
to craft a uniquely compelling story about a liberal white
woman—and a racially segregated town—both seeking to
navigate their way through the shadow of Jim Crow and the
turbulence of the Deep South in the late 1960s."

HOLLIS R. TOWNS is a writer, editor and diversity leader. He most recently
was VP of Local News for Gannett/ USA Today network.

We hold these truths to be self-evident,

that all men are created equal,

that they are endowed by their Creator

with certain unalienable Rights,

that among these are Life, Liberty and

the pursuit of Happiness.

THE DECLARATION OF INDEPENDENCE

LOOKING
for
JAZZ

*A Memoir about the Black College
and Southern Town
That Changed My Life*

ANNA R. HOLLOWAY

In memory of Miss Elaine Douglas
and Mrs. Ida Miller

Contents

PROLOGUE.

1967: The Fight for Peace and Freedom

I WAITED AT MY DESK in Karl Kroeber's Victorian Literature class for the professor to arrive, ready to take some notes. I thought I took better ones than those smart Long Islanders in the class because for me, Professor Kroeber's way of thinking just clicked.

Then we heard it. Outside, below our Bascom Hall classroom window, the usual chanting turned to yelling and screams. We ran to the window and looked down to see police beating protestors with sticks as they emerged from the doors of the Dow Building. Students in jeans, and some in military jackets, were dragged to a police van while other students jeered and yelled waving protest signs.

We thought nonviolent demonstrations were supposed to be peaceful. Anger rose up inside me. This wasn't fair!

Then the strange smell invaded our classroom through the open windows. The police had used tear gas to force out the remaining demonstrators and disperse the crowd. It had spread through the air. My eyes and nose began to burn. I couldn't believe we had been tear-gassed in English class.

Most everyone on the Bascom Hill side of the University of Wisconsin campus—the liberal arts side—was against the war in 1967. We believed in civil rights for black people, too, so we knew about nonviolent demonstrations and had seen demonstrators on our campus. A few weeks earlier, I saw police try to end a protest inside the Dow Building. The students fell to the floor and police carried them out from the building one-by-one to a waiting van.

Dow Chemical had funded the classroom where the demonstrations took place—the same company that manufactured Napalm to deforest areas of Vietnam. The Dow Building was a perfect target for demonstrating against the war.

• • •

Barely two years later, demonstrations became more violent in Madison, Wisconsin. The physics building on the other side of Bascom Hill was bombed by protesters and one graduate student killed.

By that time, I was more than nine hundred miles away, finding out firsthand about long-standing violations of civil and human rights in the state of Georgia, and my husband Mike was on his way to Vietnam.

1968–1969

1.
Landing in Georgia

Looking out the window of the plane as it neared Atlanta, I saw zig-zagging boundaries formed by wandering roads, rivers, and borders of fields, nothing like the regular checkerboard pattern of the Midwest I had flown over earlier. I wondered if Mike had ever flown over Georgia. He was back in Wisconsin now after taking me to the airport in Chicago. It was early August 1968, and I was going to see about a job in Fort Valley, Georgia.

From Atlanta, I flew to Macon, a medium-sized city near my destination. The small propeller plane taxied and came to a stop. I climbed down the short set of stairs and walked across the asphalt to the terminal. The woman who met me was about my height and on the heavy side. She had very curly black and gray hair and a few dark freckles.

"Mrs. Mitchell?" she said in a friendly but authoritative tone. "I'm pleased to meet you. I'm Elaine Douglas, head of English at Fort Valley State College. Welcome to Georgia! We must get your luggage. My car is parked right over there."

Miss Douglas wore an old-fashioned beige dress. I hoped my own brown and blue striped top and brown skirt had the right look for a traveler and a prospective English instructor.

I looked around the airport terminal. It had everything in one room and very few gates and ticket counters. The Oshkosh airport near my parents' home was bigger than this. Miss Douglas and I walked to the baggage claim only a few steps from the arrival gate. We retrieved my suitcase and headed out of the building.

"I understand you are from Wisconsin," she said.

"My family's been there about six years. Before that, I lived in Wheaton, Illinois," I told her.

"I'm very familiar with Wheaton," she said. "I am from Chicago, and I studied at the University of Chicago."

I remembered my dad had admired an economist at the University of Chicago.

I put my suitcase in the trunk and we got in her car. As we drove out of the parking lot, I looked around and saw one or two large business operations right across from the airport and then nothing but fields and woods.

Elaine Douglas was near sixty and I had just turned twenty-three. Yet it seemed like we clicked. We both had lived in the Chicago area. The University of Chicago and my school, the University of Wisconsin, both were highly respected. Miss Douglas was friendly and direct, and we got along from the beginning.

"I received my license last year," Miss Douglas said as she headed out.

I didn't know how to drive yet, myself.

We passed more large fields, the Vinson Valley Preserve (a whites-only park as I learned later), and more woods. She took the turns so fast that I felt myself holding on to my seat. I was on my way.

2.

Green, Neon, and Black

WE SLOWED DOWN as we drove through the City of Fort Valley. Sweet smells and humid air came in through the open car windows. Looking out, I saw trees, bushes, and vines with fat leaves crowding up against the sides of the brick and frame houses, not something I'd been used to seeing in the North. Block pillars held up some of the houses. I remembered a boy from Alabama in my seventh-grade class who told us houses in the South were set on blocks, not on slabs or above basements like in the North.

We rode past large historical homes and on through the intersection of the downtown where the brick, two-story buildings with store fronts below looked like the stores in most small towns I'd seen. Then we turned and went across the tracks. It was hot, the air so thick and heavy it seemed hard to breathe.

I really didn't know much about the South. The girls I played with when I was little liked General Robert E. Lee, and especially his horse, Traveler. In junior high, a girl who had moved to Wheaton from South Carolina had a charming drawl and made it seem like the South was a lovely place. But by this time, we were seeing black children on TV being escorted by police into schools while angry white adults yelled at them. Our teachers and parents taught us that segregation was wrong.

In college, I read Flannery O'Connor's *Wise Blood* with its eccentric characters and Tennessee Williams's *Cat on a Hot Tin Roof.* I looked at the pictures in Michael Harrington's *The Other America* of poor families in overalls, white and black, sitting on porches of shacks or standing beside their mules, I learned about the poverty brought about by land erosion in the largely rural and agricultural South. Still, I did not have a clear picture in my mind of the southern United States.

I came to Georgia to interview for a college teaching job — my first one — within 100 miles of Fort Benning where Mike would start his two-year Army Reserve commitment. I had my master's degree, and the United States was still entangled in the War in Vietnam. I wanted to start my teaching career near Mike.

A yellow neon sign arched over the entrance to the campus. It read FORT VALLEY STATE COLLEGE. That was different. Before this, I'd been on the campuses of Wheaton College, Ripon College, Carlton College, Oshkosh State College, and the University of Wisconsin both in Madison and in Milwaukee. They had traditional granite, brick, even concrete pillars — no neon advertising anywhere let alone at the entrances.

Fat green shrubbery grew up to the windows and at the doors of each building. And the campus was flat.

"Here is our campus. The students call it 'The Yard,'" Miss Douglas said.

I associated that term with prisons.

The road we drove in on extended all the way to the back of the campus, almost to the new stadium and the new gym. We stopped at the Lottie L. Lyons Student Center, a contemporary red brick building with some pale tan pebble-filled concrete sections under the big windows on the front and one side.

"We have a room for you here," Miss Douglas said.

She parked at the side of the building and opened the trunk so I could get my suitcase. Since I had no previous experience with professional interviews, staying on the campus for my first one did not strike me as odd.

At Oshkosh State and UW, where I had gone to college, the student unions had eating areas with booths, dining rooms, recreation rooms, TV rooms and meeting rooms. The UW Rathskeller even had a counter where we could buy 3.2 beer. All I could see here were a snack bar with a short-order kitchen at the back, a bookstore and post office on one side, and a broad expanse of floor surrounded by pillars holding up a second-story mezzanine. A few tables and chairs in front of the snack bar and under the mezzanine seemed to be the only student gathering place. It turned out the Lyons Student Center did have a small lounge and a small TV room as well as pool and ping-pong tables, but they were not visible as I walked in, and I didn't see them until much later.

We climbed straight up the stairs to the left of the snack bar and went down a short hall. The rooms here opened to look out over the railing. Miss Douglas gave me my key, and when we went in, I saw that it had a bedroom and a bathroom, like in a hotel.

"You can get ready and rest a few minutes. I'll come back in an hour to take you to your interview with the dean," Miss Douglas said.

Years later, it dawned on me that these hotel rooms were needed because black people weren't welcome at most motels and hotels in 1968.

I sat down on the bed and thought about all I'd seen so far. All the people on the campus — students walking around, staff members in the student center — were black, and, evidently, Miss Douglas also was black. I hadn't recognized that when I first saw her. We had few black students at the University of Wisconsin and none in Oshkosh. Two black student athletes who went to my Wheaton high school in Illinois had darker complexions than Miss Douglas's. I had heard of one black college, Howard University. But sitting in our apartment back in Madison searching for college teaching positions in Georgia, I didn't realize that some of the colleges I applied to were all black.

The last I heard, all public schools in the United States were supposed to be integrated according to the 1954 court order of Brown v. Board of Education, starting with first grade. We thought that sounded like a reasonable plan. I'd never even thought about integration of state colleges. Before long, I'd learn that, in Georgia, the court order simply had not been obeyed. Beginning in 1965, a very few black students had begun attending public elementary and high schools under the designation of "freedom of choice" or the "free transfer plan." And the school districts allowed only a handful of black students to attend the previously segregated white schools under this plan. The white state colleges and universities were not integrated at all.

Growing up, I'd lived in Waterville, Ohio; Wayzata, Minnesota; State College, Pennsylvania; Brookfield and Wheaton, Illinois; Oshkosh and Madison, Wisconsin. But until the year I went to Madison, my experiences were limited and close to home with my family. Now I might be on my own in a completely new place.

This is really interesting! I realized, sitting there. *Mike thinks I'm naive and I haven't been exposed to much. This could be a completely new experience—and I'll bet I'll get a chance to hear jazz, too. If I get a job here, he won't be able to say I'm naïve anymore.*

3.

"How you doin'?"

I N AN HOUR, Miss Douglas came to get me, and we walked to
a building at the front of the campus near the main entrance.

"Your interview is with Dr. Banks, the Academic Dean," Miss
Douglas said. "We call this the Carnegie Building. It once was the
library. Andrew Carnegie donated libraries to a number of small
colleges."

Inside the small red brick building, we went up the stairs to the
dean's outer office.

"This is Mrs. Mitchell," she said to the secretary seated at a desk
by the door. "She is interviewing for our instructor's position."

"Mrs. Mitchell," Miss Douglas said, turning to me, "this is Miss
Louise Chisholm, Dr. Banks' secretary."

I said hello in a polite voice.

Miss Chisholm, a dark, strong-looking woman dressed in a dark
jacket and white blouse, looked tall even sitting at her desk.

"How're you doin', Miss Mitchell? Welcome to Fort Valley!" she
said.

I said, "Thank you."

Miss Douglas left, and it was quiet for a minute.

"It doesn't get this hot very often where I come from," I said,
making conversation.

"Shu-ut up!" said Miss Chisholm. "Where you from?"

"Ohio, Minnesota, Pennsylvania, Illinois, and Wisconsin," came
my stock answer.

"Shu-ut up!" Miss Chisholm said.

Then Dr. Banks indicated that he was ready, and Miss Chisholm ushered me into his office.

"Welcome to The Fort Valley State College," Dr. Banks said in the mellowest, deepest possible voice. I noted his very dark brown complexion and small amount of black hair. Many years later when I edited his memoir, *Up from the 'Sip*, I learned that he came from the Delta region where Mississippi and Louisiana come together, and he was educated by Quakers in Ohio. Before becoming dean, he was a sociology professor.

"The position we have open for an English instructor is a Woodrow Wilson Teaching Fellowship," Dr. Banks explained. "It is for one year, and it pays $4000. You would be teaching four three-hour classes each quarter."

He smiled at me, showing his white teeth.

I nodded. I'd been proud since childhood that my father had taught in college at Penn State. "My father used to be a college professor," I would tell people. He had returned to the profession when I was sixteen and now taught economics, marketing, and sales at Oshkosh State College.

In spite of this and my years as a college and university student, I didn't understand academic rank. But I had passed my masters comps and since I was not required to write a thesis for my program at the University of Wisconsin, I met the qualifications to be a college instructor. Now I could follow in my dad's footsteps.

"How did you come to be interested in this position?" asked Dr. Banks.

"I got my degrees so I could teach English in college," I responded. "I've always liked writing and literature. I applied in Georgia to be near my husband who is going for training at Fort Benning."

"I believe you will find the Fort Valley State College and our students to be welcoming," he said.

After we had more pleasant conversation, Dr. Banks concluded, "Thank you for coming, hear? You should be receiving a letter or phone call from us very soon if we are able to hire you for the position."

Miss Douglas was waiting in Miss Chisholm's office.

"How did you like Dr. Banks?" she asked.

"He is very nice," I said. "He said I will hear from him soon."

"Now let's go to the English office," she said, "and we can talk about what you will teach if you are offered the position and you accept."

We walked to the larger red brick building next door, what was then called the Academic Building and now is Founders Hall. I noticed the tall cupola on top with a clock on its front. Inside, I saw tall ceilings but noticed that the woodwork was not as beautiful as Carnegie's.

"This building and several others at the front of the campus were built with student labor," Miss Douglas told me. "They include the Ohio Hall dormitory, Huntington Hall, Patton Hall, which is the music building, and Bishop, the dining hall."

She sat behind her desk when we went into her small office. The dark reddish wood furniture looked old and mismatched. Her desk had several piles of paper on it. I could see at least three bookcases crammed with books behind her. "What did you study in college and graduate school?" she asked after I sat down facing her.

Miss Douglas rubbed her mouth, and I noticed a little moustache. I also noticed the high waist of her light brown dress above her stomach. But I felt nothing but respect for her. My mind was focused on giving a strong impression of myself as a potential college instructor.

"Most of my graduate classes were in British literature, plus I had one linguistics class," I answered. "I did have a good cultural American history class as a senior that included literature. And we studied American plays in my honors seminar."

We did not concentrate on one area of literature for our master's at Wisconsin in the late sixties. I had classes on subjects ranging from Chaucer's *Canterbury Tales* in the Middle Ages to E.M. Forster's *Howard's End*, James Joyce's *Portrait of an Artist*, and Virginia Woolf's *Mrs. Dalloway*, novels written in the beginning of the twentieth century. The comprehensive exam covered all the areas in British literature, including my weak area, Old English.

"Presently," Miss Douglas said, "our majors receive a degree that lists them as having a major in secondary education with a concentration in English. I do hope to develop a pure English major, a baccalaureate in English. Would you like to work on that?"

"I really would!" I said.

By this time, we were ready to eat dinner. Miss Douglas invited me to ride with her to the Dairy Queen. They served us from a window, and we ate our hamburgers and fries in the car.

In fact, Fort Valley didn't have any sit-down restaurants on the white side of town in 1968 that I can remember. Instead, they had family-style dining rooms in some private homes. The black side of town had a café, the Shrimp Boat, and the College Inn although Miss Douglas didn't choose to take me to one of them.

The next morning, I came down the marble stairs from my room up on the mezzanine and walked over to the snack bar. It smelled like bacon. As I came up to the rather high counter to order breakfast, I saw a big refrigerator, a big griddle, pots and pans, and cooking supplies such as containers of shortening behind the counter. The snack bar ladies and student workers wore white paper caps like shower caps over their hair, and they smiled at me.

"Hi," I said.

"Fine, thank you. I'm doin' good," said the lady behind the counter.

It took me a minute to realize that my "Hi" was interpreted as "How are you?"

"How you doin' this morning?" the snack bar lady asked.

I didn't know I was supposed to say, "Fine, thank you."

So I said, "I'm doing okay, thanks."

"'Tin I help you?" she asked.

I asked for a fried egg, over easy, and bacon. I got white bread buttered and browned on the griddle on one side, grits with some margarine on them, eggs, and strips of bacon, all on a wobbly paper plate with a plastic fork.

I carried my breakfast over to one of the snack bar tables to eat, thinking about the fact that my mom only gave us grits when we had fried ham and red-eye gravy.

From my table near the door, I looked out at the wide expanse of the tiled student center floor.

Why is the floor so big and empty? I wondered.

A few students sat in wood cubby holes outside of the bookstore. Others walked around the edges of the floor. I thought the few who walked across looked self-conscious on the open floor in front of everybody.

I know I'd be self-conscious, I said to myself. The anomaly of the large, empty student center floor stayed on my mind.

After I ate my breakfast, I got my luggage out of the room and met Miss Douglas back downstairs where I gave her my key.

Soon I was on my way back to meet Mike at the airport in Chicago. Sitting on the plane, I went over my new experiences. I would have to tell Mike all about it. Then I would wait for a letter or call.

4.

Shakespeare and Ammo

MIKE WAS WAITING for me at the gate when I came off the plane from Atlanta. His hair, lighter than mine, looked especially blonde. His stance and his shoulders showed the work he had been doing with his weights.

"How'd it go?" he asked, giving me a hug before he picked up my suitcase.

"It's a black college," I said. I had seen the black staff, students, and faculty members, but I'm sure it seemed abstract to him. "I think I might get the job. When are you supposed to report to Fort Benning?"

"September 15," he answered. "If you get the job, we're going to need a moving van."

We drove back to Madison in the red Dodge Dart his mother gave us after she got a new car, speculating about where to live. Mike must have been visualizing his jump school and Ranger training while I thought about teaching in those red brick buildings.

Two letters came in a few days. One, from Dr. Banks, offered me the Woodrow Wilson Teaching Fellowship and instructor position at Fort Valley State College. The other contained an offer from Tuskegee Institute, another black college.

The fellowship to teach at Fort Valley was federally funded. I didn't know what to make of that. Also, though I had gone to two state schools for my undergraduate and graduate education, I had always been attracted to private schools. As a private school, Tuskegee could have been appealing, but just that summer, a taxi driver had been shot during a civil rights protest there. Tuskegee, Alabama, sounded dangerous.

Anyway, I hadn't seen Tuskegee or met anyone there. I liked Miss Douglas and I had seen the Fort Valley campus. I accepted the offer from Fort Valley State College and didn't look back.

Like many baby-boomers, I opposed the draft and the military action in Vietnam. Mike said he agreed with me. He'd only joined the Reserve Officer Training Corps to keep from being drafted after his grades went down. But he loved guns—although he'd shot himself in the leg while practicing quick-draws, and he devoted hours to reloading ammunition. He also idolized an uncle who had been a soldier in World War II. The idea of becoming a second lieutenant in the infantry, a paratrooper, and a Ranger excited him.

The Monday after we got back to our apartment on the south side of Madison, Wisconsin, I took a city bus downtown, got off at the end of State Street, and climbed the hill to Bascom Hall. Passing the statue of Abraham Lincoln at the front of the building where I had sat in so many English and history classes, I went inside to the third floor graduate office of the English Department, the one for master's candidates. I planned to announce proudly to the master's program director, Standish Henning, that I had secured a college teaching position. He always told us to try teaching before deciding whether to go on for the PhD to be sure we wouldn't end up studying years for a career we didn't like. Now I was doing just that.

He invited me into his office where I looked around at the fine old office furniture and his Shakespeare and Renaissance books on the shelves. I had taken one Shakespeare class from Mr. Henning, and the other from the most famous English scholar at the University of Wisconsin, Madeline Doran, a literary critic and a poet.

From Mr. Henning's window, I could see down to the foot of Bascom Hill to State Street and some of the restaurants, stores, and bars I frequented as a student.

Mr. Henning had short reddish hair and wore eyeglasses, and a tweed jacket.

"I wanted to tell you that I interviewed at Fort Valley State College in Georgia," I began, "and I have received an offer to work as an instructor there. I'm getting a Woodrow Wilson Fellowship. It's a black college, like Howard."

I waited, expecting his congratulations.

"Perhaps you should keep looking," Mr. Henning responded. "If you start by taking this position, your promising career as an academic will effectively be over."

I left his office stunned and deflated. I wouldn't get prestige if I took the job! On the bus ride home, I weighed the situation.

It didn't matter, I decided. With Mike about to continue his military training and go to Vietnam, I had more than my distant future career to think about. His degrees from Kenyon College, The University of the South (Sewanee), and Harvard University would not have acquainted him with black Americans, let alone black colleges.

When I got back to our apartment, I heard, "Chunk, bang. Chunk, chunk, bang."

Mike was busy reloading ammunition, or ammo, as he called it, at the long, red-painted desk we'd created by combining a bedside chest of drawers and a small desk. I didn't know which one of his guns the ammo was for since I didn't really care for guns.

"Do you know what Mr. Henning said?" I asked as I came in.

"What?" asked Mike, pausing his reloading.

"He said if I take this position, my career is practically over."

"I'll tell him, 'Look Jack, don't you know there's a war going on?'" Mike responded.

"We've got more on our minds than picking a status school for me to work at," I agreed. "I just got my master's, for crying out loud."

Our young cats, Mr. Fu (Lai Fu) and Pokey, were playing around the small second floor apartment. We had a living room, a kitchen, a bathroom, and one bedroom. Mr. Fu was trying to climb the curtains in the living room again.

I went into the kitchen to work on dinner.

"You know what I've always wanted?" I called into the other room. "A mobile home. I think trailers are neat. They have everything you need, all organized and put together. It's like when Nancy and I used to play cowboys. She had little plastic figures of Roy Rogers and Dale Evans, and I had a red rubber motorcycle man I named Jack that I got from my cousin Larry's old toys. We had fun using dollhouse furniture, little fences, lots of wood blocks, and little boxes to make houses and corrals for them."

"Yeah?" said Mike.

"Fixing up a mobile home so we make good use of the space in it would be sort of like playing cowboys in real life. Anyway, you'll be going different places. Maybe I'll only work there a year or half a year, and then we could have the trailer moved to the next place you'll be stationed."

"I don't know anything about you and your sister's cowboys. I played with cap guns and bikes. But it's not a bad idea," Mike answered from the other room.

After I had formally accepted the job, Miss Douglas wrote and offered to help us find a place to stay in Fort Valley. She seemed very receptive to the idea of a mobile home and offered to help us get a lot in a park to set it up. I didn't understand until later that no one in the white community would rent to a white person who worked at the college so that having our own mobile home on the side of town near the campus was a very good idea.

Mike and I began looking up companies that sold mobile homes. One of them had a factory in Valdosta, Georgia, and could deliver the mobile home to Fort Valley. We chose the model named "Buddy" and placed our order. Buddy was white with blue trim and was twelve feet wide and fifty feet long. The lot we were instructed to have it delivered to was on Dr. Houston Stallworth's property a little outside the City of Fort Valley and a mile from the campus.

5.

Farewell

IN THE APARTMENT kitchen of Ruth and Buck Anderson, our friends in Madison, Ruth and I were getting the food ready to put on the table. It was a going away supper for Mike and me. Bob Ayanian and Susie Bible were there, too.

"I'll help slice the tomatoes," I offered.

Ruth looked at what I was doing and said, "Always cut out the stem area before you slice a tomato."

"Okay," I said, making a note to myself. Preoccupied with my coming job, I said, "You and Buck are both from Texas. Are there black colleges in Texas?"

"I can think of Paul Quinn, Prairie View, and Texas Southern," Ruth answered. "I'm sure you'll like it fine."

"They're not just in the South," she continued. She was a journalist, doing graduate work in the field, and she had a reservoir of information. "There's Lincoln in Pennsylvania and Central in Ohio, for example. I think there are over a hundred of those schools, all told."

"I don't think most people realize that," I said, "at least up here. Are many of them private instead of state?" I'd dreamed of being at a small private school since my visit to Carlton College during my sophomore year at Oshkosh State College. Then I chose the University of Wisconsin to be with Mike.

"Some are," she said.

Even Oshkosh State was bigger than Fort Valley State College. I grew up living in middle-sized cities, State College, Wheaton, and Oshkosh. I thought about riding past the stores and the old houses in Fort Valley, over the tracks, and past the really small houses on the way to campus. I had one thing going for me, I thought. I knew about coming to new places and fitting in.

We crowded around the kitchen table at supper, and Buck told us about the science fiction novel he was sending out for publication.

"I'm going to read *Stranger in a Strange Land* by Robert Heinlein," I said. "Is your book sort of like that?"

Buck laughed. "Yeah, if you add in Texas Rangers and some serious chase scenes! I'll let you know when it comes out."

As I listened to Buck, I thought, not for the first time, that he looked like the actor Fess Parker who played Davy Crockett on television. Buck had gone to prison rather than be drafted or escape to Canada, which was impressive to me, but hard to imagine, even though I was against the draft and the war.

"When I publish, it won't be that exciting," Bob said. "I just got the letter I've been waiting for — I got into grad school at the University of Southern California. People think USC is a state school since California is in its name and it's big, but it's private."

Bob was slimmer and less macho than Buck, reflecting his Armenian heritage.

"I'm going to study econometrics," he told us. His girlfriend Susie looked a little sad, and I wondered if she was going to California with him. A Madison native, she was much younger than her boyfriend and slim, with long medium-brown hair, straight and silky smooth.

I looked at Mike.

"I want to go into film production. After these next two years are over," he said.

We all felt anxiety about his going to Vietnam. I started getting migraine headaches if we went to the movies. The bright lights and loud sounds of movies triggered the headaches and nausea, but my constant worry must have made me susceptible.

Somehow, from among the thousands of students at the University of Wisconsin, Ruth and Buck, Bob and Susie, and Mike and I had found each other and bonded as friends.

And like so many in our generation, I had started to question traditional social rules. My parents would not have approved, to put it mildly, but Mike and I started living together near the end of our first year in Madison, in the beginning of 1966, even though our wedding was not until the summer of 1967. After we were married Mike went to Advanced Camp, and we rented an apartment upstairs in a private home. But our kittens running up and down the hall bothered the owners, and we were told to leave. We got our second apartment that fall, Mike finished his last few classes, and I began my coursework for the master's degree.

Now we were leaving that apartment. After our supper and more talk with our friends, we said goodbye to them, feeling both anticipation and sadness.

With our mobile home scheduled to arrive in Fort Valley, we packed our things into a moving van, put Pokey and Lai Fu into a cat carrier, and set off for Georgia.

When we stopped and got a motel on the south side of Atlanta, Pokey hid under the bed, and Lai Fu had a great time climbing the carpeted walls.

6.

Snakes and Neighbors

MIKE AND I both blinked. We'd just seen a little rattler wriggle away from the grassy space in the lot where our mobile home was being hooked up.

"Just take a look-see before you step," Dr. Stallworth said cheerfully.

Dr. Houston Stallworth, our new landlord, wore a short-sleeved white dress shirt and a dark tie.

"I teach and do research in Agriculture," he said. "This property around my house has got setups for about ten mobile homes, five on the side where your home is going, and five on the dirt road next to me, behind the house a ways. You get electric, water, sewer, and you can pay for propane."

"We did order a gas stove," I said. "That's what I'm used to, so I'm glad there's propane."

"Don't think there'll be too many more snakes. But keep your eyes open. Most of them not poisonous. I keep a rat snake in my kitchen cupboard for mice. Rat snakes aren't poisonous, in case you see one. They're long and black."

I noticed that Dr. Stallworth, sort of like Miss Douglas, had loosely curled black hair (hers was salt and pepper), and, like her, he had a light complexion, especially compared with Dr. Banks and Miss Chisholm and the snack bar staff. He wore dark-rimmed glasses and had a smile most of the time.

The white frame house he lived in was set on blocks and had a small, covered porch. We saw fields across the street and woods on both sides of the Stallworth property and in the back.

The living room end of our new trailer faced South Macon Street (now State University Drive). Just a short distance down the way, the street became an unpaved red dirt road—red clay. At that point it became the Old Marshallville Road.

A utility pole already stood at the other end of our home, and a propane tank near that, on the side. Our mobile home had visible wheels with cement blocks to hold it up, and we stacked more of the blocks to serve as the steps to our back door. A set of wood steps on a metal frame served as the front doorsteps—the "stoop," as they called it.

"Look, Mike," I said after Dr. Stallworth welcomed us to Georgia again and said goodbye. "Some of our neighbors are coming to meet us."

I said, "Hello!" and Mike said "Hey!" as they walked toward us.

"We the Henrys," the rather short woman said. "How you doin'?"

"Fine, thanks, how are you?" I answered, having learned by now that this was the expected greeting.

"You goin' to work at the college?" Maybelle wanted to know. "Mr. Henry, he work over there. He a security guard," she said.

Mr. Henry, a big man, looked over at us and down at his wife, smiled, and remained silent. I noticed that both were on the dark side, though not as dark as Dr. Banks.

"I'm going to teach English at the college," I answered. We swatted at gnats as we talked.

"We been here two years," Maybelle volunteered. "We come from the coast, near to Brunswick."

Her accent differed from Dr. Stallworth's and that of other people I'd met so far on campus, but I didn't have any trouble understanding her.

"We moved here from Wisconsin," I replied, not wanting to go into my usual "Ohio, Minnesota, Pennsylvania, Illinois, and Wisconsin" routine.

"I thought maybe you was from Minnesota like those college students who come down last year for the vote," said Maybelle.

She turned out to be the first of many who thought I'd come directly out of Minnesota like the voter registration volunteers in Peach County the year before. It was no wonder, since I had blondish hair and looked young enough to be a college student. And I was from Minnesota on my father's side.

"You come see us, hear?" Maybelle invited us.

By this time, their two children, a boy about six or seven and a girl about four, were playing around her legs.

"Take Sister back to the house," she told the boy. "You bad!"

I didn't think he was being very bad, and I didn't think people should tell their children that, but he did seem active.

After the movers—both the mobile home transport men and the men with the moving van—had driven away, Mike and I got into the Dodge Dart and headed downtown to look around and buy food and gas.

"There's a Gulf station. We can pull in there," I said after we'd crossed the tracks and were in the center of town.

Under the big, round orange Gulf sign, we read the words, "Smisson's Gulf." In those days, gas station attendants came up, pumped your gas, cleaned your windshield, offered to check your oil, and chatted while the gas flowed into the car.

"How you doin'?" asked the short and stocky man at our window. "I'm Buddy Smisson, owner of this here station. I see y'all from Wisconsin. How you all happen to come this way?"

"I'm going to be teaching at the college," I answered.

"What do your mother and father think about that?"

"Oh, our parents know we're moving here," I said.

After a pause, and with a note of resignation, he said, "Welp. It's coming."

In a polite manner, with no noticeable hostility, he was referring to integration—in this case, white integration of a black school. I think he asked the question about our parents because he probably understood people based on their families.

A lot has changed in Fort Valley, mostly for the better. But when it comes to the integration of communities, I still have to say, "It's coming."

After buying food for dinner at the Colonial Store, we parked the car in the trailer park's central driveway away from South Macon Street and went inside our brand-new living room where the movers had placed our black Naugahyde sofa that opened up to serve as our bed.

I set the groceries on the Formica counter and put some in the refrigerator and some in the wood cabinets above the counter.

Mike gave me an embrace from behind, then went to organize his weights and reloading equipment in the first small bedroom.

My sewing machine and the big yellow trunk holding my fabric were in the room at the end.

The living room carpet, in avocado green, contrasted with the brand-new copper-colored kitchen appliances and the Philippine mahogany paneling around the good-sized living room, down the hall and in all the other rooms except the bathroom. We put the red-painted desk in the first room, and it wasn't long before I could hear Mike back reloading his ammo. I had my clothes and my green desk in the last room along with the trunk filled with sewing supplies and fabric. A floral Japanese paper lantern finished it off. Before long, I would sew rich colored pink, red, blue, and green flowered curtains for all the windows.

"Let's get boards and bricks to make shelves for all our books," I called back to Mike.

I felt nervous but ready. My job as an English instructor and his as an Army officer lay before us.

7.

Collard Greens and
Teachers' Desks

I LOOKED IN THE MIRROR at the light blue, store-bought dress I put on to wear to the faculty dinner. The dinner was a ritual the week before classes at Fort Valley State College in those days.

"Does this look ok?" I asked Mike on our way down the back steps headed for the car.

"Looks great to me," he said.

He drove me down the road about a mile to the campus, turned under the neon arch, and let me off close to Bishop, the dining hall. "Good luck!" he said.

Bishop Hall was only one story, not two like the other red brick buildings nearby. Long tables filled the large, open room. A serving line in the back normally handled the students. But for this beginning of the year faculty dinner, it looked like we would be served at our places.

My seat at one of the tables faced the back wall and serving line. I saw an older lady back there who seemed to be managing things.

"That's Miss Junia Fambro. She doesn't just provide meals. She makes sure the students learn their manners," said the man sitting next to me. "She'll scold them or put them out if they don't behave and try to learn proper etiquette."

He got quiet then as we were about to say a prayer to bless the food and the new school year.

When the prayer finished, student dining hall workers began placing plates full of food before all the seated faculty members. I looked at the plate in front of me and saw a half a Cornish game hen with rice and a very thoroughly cooked green vegetable. The only greens I knew about were spinach and Swiss chard.

"What kind of vegetable is this?" I asked.

"I'm George Holland, in music," he introduced himself, reaching for a little glass bottle containing small, light green peppers and a light-colored liquid. "Those are collards, and we like to put this pepper sauce on them."

"Oh, I'm Anna Mitchell. I'm going to teach English."

The watery pepper sauce had a slightly hot flavor. It was good on the greens.

I changed schools so often growing up, I learned to be sociable with everyone when I come to a new situation. Only time will tell which of the people might become my friends. As I had done all those other times when I moved to new places or started in new schools, I looked around the room at all the people I hadn't gotten to know yet. Practically everyone in this room was black. I did see a few people who seemed to be from India as well as maybe three or four white faces.

"Department meetings will take place tomorrow morning," Dean Banks announced as the dinner ended. "Full faculty meetings normally take place at seven PM on Fridays in the Hunt Library. However, the first full faculty meeting of this new school year will be at two o'clock the day after tomorrow following the orientation and luncheon at the President's house for our new faculty members."

Mike waited to pick me up after the dinner. I told him the banquet was fine. When we got back to Buddy the mobile home, Mike went into his little room for a while to reload ammo, and I heard the familiar, "Chunk! Chunk! Bang!"

I went to my room and looked in my closet to decide what dress or skirt and blouse to wear to the English faculty meeting.

My department met the next day on the first floor of the Academic Building in an office with room for about ten faculty members.

"This desk will be yours," Miss Douglas told me, and she pointed to an old brown desk right in the middle of the room.

"Thank you," I said, and I sat down.

I could tell the office used to be a classroom because a blackboard filled the wall that we faced—what would have been the front of a class. To my right, a series of tall windows let the light in through disorderly venetian blinds that looked like they would be hard to raise or lower. The hardwood floor looked old, too, uneven and clean but not shiny.

The other faculty members' desks were similar in size to mine, and each, like mine, had a chair for students next to it. Different finishes and details on the desks showed some were older than others and they must have been brought in from different locations. To my left, against the wall by the door, stood three modest bookshelves filled with books and stacks of paper. The shelves looked hand-made, maybe by workers at the college. Decor wasn't a priority here, but it wasn't in most English offices I'd visited in Wisconsin, either, although each faculty member there had his own office. (They all were men.)

I didn't find myself thinking about being the only white person in the room, probably because I could see the others, but I couldn't see myself. Miss Douglas came to the front of the room, taking over Mrs. Cook's desk and facing us.

"Colleagues," she began, "I'm pleased to introduce Mrs. Anna Mitchell who will be teaching English with us this year. Mrs. Mitchell is from Wisconsin and has just earned her master's degree. Please join me in welcoming her."

After a bit of applause, each person welcomed me, going in order around the room: Mrs. Delores Cook, Mrs. Sadie Malone, Mr. Joseph McGhee, Mr. JC Hill, Mrs. Doris Adams, Miss Alma Jan Green, Mr. Joseph Adkins, Mr. Ellis Hunter, and Mrs. Louise Powell. Each said a few words except Mr. McGhee who only gave me a shy nod.

At twenty-three, I was the youngest; and at the level of instructor, I had the lowest rank. No one in the department had a PhD or even an EdD, so we all were Mrs., Miss, Ms, or Mr.

I had plenty of confidence. Probably too much. I believed I was ready to share my knowledge with students.

"Please have your course outlines ready by the first day of class," Miss Douglas said. "I won't read the list, but we have new textbooks for Freshman English and Introduction to Literature. Please get your copies from Mrs. Jones and refer to them in your syllabi. Mrs. Mitchell, you will be teaching the first part of Survey of English Literature, and Mrs. Jones has a copy of that book for you, as well."

"Mrs. Jones can help you use the mimeograph machine if you type your syllabus on one of those stencils," Mrs. Adams shared with me in a low voice. "If you want to write out a syllabus or handout by hand, you can use a Thermofax master. The Thermofax machine is in the back or the room, over there."

She pointed to a machine on a little table at the back between the big windows and the door to the room.

"Some people make Mrs. Jones type them," Mrs. Adams added with a wry smile, "but I think she has enough to do to help Miss Douglas. We all ought to know how to type." She cast a significant look over at Mrs. Malone.

Miss Douglas chose what turned out to be excellent texts to guide us in our teaching and, in a sense, to teach me how to teach English. I still have my copies of most of those books.

Back at our mobile home that night, I made spaghetti with meat sauce for Mike and me and told him about the English faculty and the faculty office.

"I'm going to see the whole faculty tomorrow afternoon," I told him. "But first, they said there's an orientation for new faculty. You can take me to the campus at ten o'clock for that. Then, we're supposed to have a luncheon at President Blanchet's house."

"Are you scared?" Mike asked.

"No, just curious. I don't think I have to talk or anything."

8.
No More In Loco Parentis

"PLEASE STAND closer together," said Mr. Maddox, the photographer, adjusting our positions with his hand by turning some people and moving some closer together so everyone would be seen in the picture.

We, the new Fort Valley State College faculty members, stood on the front steps of the Hunt Library (named the Bywaters Building today). We'd just finished a short orientation session learning about the academic calendar, when and where we would be paid, something called the Scope Chart, and where to find the Registrar's office and other important offices. One at a time, we'd stood and introduced ourselves. The new agriculture faculty included Dr. Ronald Abe, a short of stature Japanese man from Hilo, Hawaii, with a PhD in Animal Science from Kansas State, and Dr. Syed Raman, in plant science, from India. Clovis Tanner, a tall, white southerner, was a French instructor. Dr. Geoffrey Ibim, from Nigeria by way of Cambridge University in the UK, was an education professor. Jeffrey Way, from Ohio and then New York City University, would teach art. Scott Lewis and I were English instructors. He was from Vanderbilt and would be teaching in the College Educational Achievement Program (CEAP), so his desk was not in the same office as mine. Altogether, there were ten new faculty members in the fall of 1968, all from different places. I tried to form impressions of the other new colleagues based on where they were from.

"So, you have a masters in English from Wisconsin?" Scott asked me after the photographer was through. "I just got mine from Vanderbilt."

"Robert Penn Warren was there," I somehow happened to remember.

"Yes, we're known for creative writing," Scott replied. "So far, I'm only studying writing, not doing it myself."

"I didn't see you at the English Department meeting," I said.

"I'm in a different program," Scott started to explain. Then he was interrupted by the Asian looking Ron Abe who was in Agriculture.

"I live next to Scott," Ron said. "We have rooms in Stokey's."

"It's a small apartment house at the edge of the campus on South Macon Street," Scott explained. "It's not much of a building. Ron, here, took two of my cat's kittens," he added. "My cat's a Siamese, but their daddy definitely isn't. The kittens are sleek like Siamese, but they're all black. I see Ron likes to play fight with them. Not a good idea. They might be dangerous when they get bigger!"

"Their back arch and their tail get big," Ron explained with a funny smile. "I never had cats before. You know anything about Stokey? I hear he's in prison."

"I think that's a rumor about Stokey in prison," said Scott.

"No," I answered. "I don't know anything about that." I couldn't picture the apartment they were talking about. But I was glad to hear about the cats.

Before we could introduce ourselves further, Mrs. Maude Black, the president's secretary, said, "Come, everyone. It's time to go to Dr. Blanchet's home for the luncheon,"

"We can go together in my car," Scott offered, so we left the library steps and headed in his car down South Macon Street to a neighborhood with brick ranch style houses.

During lunch, which consisted of iced tea, little salads, and sandwiches with the crusts cut off, I told Ron and Scott and others, including Jeff Way and Clovis Tanner who were sitting nearby, about my husband.

"In about two weeks, Mike has to report to Fort Benning for jump school and Ranger training," I said.

"That's outside of Columbus, near Alabama," Clovis Tanner interjected in his mellow southern drawl. "About a hundred miles from here, I think."

"You need ride to school, Scott and I can bring you," offered Ron. And that is how our friendship began.

After lunch, we had to go back to the campus and to the second floor in the Hunt Library for the general faculty meeting. We took seats together toward the back.

"The meeting will come to order," said Dr. Blanchet.

I noted that Dr. Banks was W.S.M. Banks and Dr. Blanchet was W.W.E. Blanchet, but I didn't know what all those initials stood for. In fact, Dr. Blanchet was Waldo and Dr. Banks was William, affectionately referred to as Bill. The slight and light-skinned Dr. Blanchet, graduate of another black college, Talladega, had earned his masters and PhD in chemistry at the University of Michigan. He addressed us with the demeanor of a true gentleman and earned my respect from the beginning. I don't know whether he actually was president-elect at that time rather than president since his inauguration, modest compared to those that came after, took place in the form of a banquet later my first year. But he was introduced as our president and served in that position during my entire first four years at Fort Valley State.

Dr. Blanchet spoke calmly at this, my first general faculty meeting, and the first meeting of the school year. But several of the faculty members stood up to speak in loud and contentious tones. I confess that, at later meetings, I raised my hand on a regular basis and stood up to make my points. I've never been shy about talking. Even though I joined this faculty at the young age of twenty-three, I thought I could contribute because I had been to other places and seen other ways of doing things. But at this first meeting, I had the sense to be quiet. I didn't even whisper comments to Ron and Scott who were sitting next to me.

"Dr. Pearson?" Dr. Blanchet called on our dean of students.

"Thank you, Dr. Blanchet," said Ozias Pearson as he stood to address the faculty.

I thought the tall Dr. Pearson, with his wavy hair, was very handsome.

"We have a new policy we must take under consideration when working with our students," Dr. Pearson said. "Traditionally, Fort Valley State College has played a role in guiding the personal lives of our students as well as their academic development. The federal government refers to this as being *in locus parentis*. The decision has come down that at the age of eighteen, students are to be considered as having the rights of adults. For that reason, we are proscribed from serving *in locus parentis* from now on. We may continue to set curfews and limits on who may enter dormitories, but aside from that, we must cease to involve the institution, as an institution, in the students' personal lives."

A somewhat portly and very plainly dressed woman on the other side of the room stood up.

"Miss Anderson?" said Dr. Blanchet.

"We have a responsibility to these young people!" she said in a strong voice. "These chil'ren going to be making babies if we don't do what is right while they are in our care!"

Miss Anderson was a college librarian, and she spent her days helping the students. I could see that she was a valiant fighter, especially for the morals and safety of young women. I thought that if the University of Wisconsin ever served *in loco parentis*, we didn't know about it. My first two years in college while attending Oshkosh State, I lived with my family a block from the campus. But when I got to Madison to attend the university, I was totally free of oversight. The private housing unit I stayed in with Luanna, my roommate from Oshkosh, must have had some rules, but we let each other in at night, as necessary. By the end of my first year there, I frequently stayed overnight in Mike's room, and she often stayed with her boyfriend also. Beginning in the summer, Mike and I moved in together. I'm fairly sure my parents didn't know of our cohabitation since I rented a room with some girls in a different apartment, my residence of record.

Today at this faculty meeting, I took in all the information presented, not realizing it portended real changes in the student experience at Fort Valley State College

9.

Thermofaxes and Alligators

M Y DESK in the middle of the large English faculty office faced Mrs. Cook's up by the blackboard. I didn't know the whole straightening process for taking care of black hair back then, but I noticed her dark hair was short to medium and turned under, what we used to call a page boy. We already had been chatting with each other.

"Mrs. Jones is good to us, and she'll help you make copies of your syllabi," Mrs. Cook said.

Then, echoing what Mrs. Adams had whispered to me in our first department meeting, she added, "Some people in the department don't want to type their own. I type mine, but I do ask her to run them off on the Mimeograph machine. There's a typewriter here in our office."

"I might do mine on my typewriter at home," I said. "I have a used Smith Corona office model that I got when I was in college. Can I do my outlines pretty much like my instructors did, mainly saying what the reading assignments are for each week?"

"That will be fine," she reassured me. "You'll need to do handouts to go with some of your lessons. It's easier to use the Thermofax machine back there for those since you can just write on the stencils and run off the copies. I'll show you. Be sure to give the dates of your tests and finals in the syllabus, though."

Our colleague JC Hill had come in during our conversation. I thought he looked a bit more dapper than the older men in the department with his curly hair and small moustache.

"Thing is to get the students to do the work," he said shaking his head. "I make 'em practice, sure do!"

Mrs. Malone was working quietly over to my right, and I noticed that she was checking back and forth with a manual while completing her outlines. From the cover, I figured out that she was working from a high school instructor's manual. I got on my high horse over that. I didn't have a good opinion of high school English compared with the courses I had in college, so I strongly disapproved. In fact, over the years I would make it a point to construct my plans for each class from scratch, referring back to notes from my own college classes as well as to the excellent textbooks Miss Douglas assigned. These books did not come with instructors' manuals.

Sometimes in my drive to be original, however, I would leave out important elements from previous quarters or semesters. Mrs. Malone may have avoided doing that.

After I finished working in the Academic Building, I went to get our mail which was delivered to the campus post office rather than to our mobile home. I turned left out of the Academic Building and walked between the Hunt Library on my left and Peabody Trades on my right. Before I got to the Lyons Student Center, I noticed something by the library that looked like a big bathtub. Curious, I stepped past some azalea bushes and across the grass to get a better look. It was a little pool, and an alligator was swimming around in it. It wasn't huge, but it wasn't small either, maybe four feet long from head to tail.

Years later, when I'd describe what I saw, people didn't believe me. Finally, I got to know Berry Jordan, a Fort Valley resident who had been raised nearby and played on the campus as a child. When I told him what I remembered, he confirmed my story. Fort Valley State College did have an alligator swimming around between two of the buildings. I still don't know why.

10.

A Sikh, the Two-Step, a Geechee, and Jazz

A FTER MIKE reported to Fort Benning for parachute training or what they called jump school, I got better acquainted with our neighbors. After Mike and I moved in, we introduced ourselves to the Jacksons whose mobile home was behind ours, but we hadn't really talked. I heard their music playing, especially in the evenings, and the beat of the bass always reminded me of a washing machine.

As I dug holes to transplant some small boxwoods, Rufus and Mary Jackson came out to see what I was doing. I had dug up the plants in the woods behind their place.

"You're making your place look good," Mary said. "We haven't bothered to do that. I'm still in college over there, you know. If we wasn't married, I'd have to stay in the dorms. Those girls have a curfew." She laughed, a deep throaty laugh, and added. "But some of those girls in the dorms let the young men in after the curfew."

I liked Mary with her low, melodious voice and amused views of things.

"You plantin' some trees?" Rufus asked. That was more than he usually said, I would learn, maybe because he had a slight lisp or a speech impediment.

"No, just shrubbery," I said. "My husband Mike is at Fort Benning now, doing training."

"We're having some friends over on Friday," Mary said. "Come on over, hear?"

Later that day, I had a conversation with Dr. Harbans Singh who lived in the mobile home next to Mary and Rufus Jackson. He introduced himself as a Sikh. He said that was why he wore a turban and didn't cut his hair and why he wore a metal bracelet. It represented a shield. Dr. Singh was an education professor and director of the Upward Bound Program for high school students preparing for college.

The people I knew from India before coming to Georgia were closer to my age and, by American standards of the time, dramatic and egotistical. Mike and I laughed about a young nan from India who spoke at Oshkosh State and used a formal British debate style to argue a conservative position. He had an accent and started each point with the proclamation, "Number One, whether or not…" "Number Two, whether or not…" and so on.

In the house where Mike and I lived together in Madison before we got married, one of our roommates was an Indian PhD student studying statistics, or as he pronounced it, "STA-tistics." He introduced himself whenever he met someone new by saying, "I am Ram Chandra Dahiya, *In*dia!"

I learned from Ram how to cook curried vegetables even though we didn't have access to ghee. We were amused by how frightened he got when tornadoes were reported on TV ("We live in Tornado Alley!") and his fear of hay fever ("Is it epidemic?").

My new Indian acquaintance, Dr. Singh, either because of his age and experience or because he was a Sikh, was calmer and more dignified.

When the Friday of the Jackson's party arrived, I crossed the small patch of weedy grass between our places and knocked on their front door. I could hear the soul music already. I didn't think of contributing beer or wine. I just brought myself. Before I knew it, Mary and Rufus were teaching me how to two-step to the sounds of Aretha, the Four Tops, and the Temptations.

At least the music wasn't new to me. Mike's parents were divorced, and he used to leave Oshkosh each summer to stay with his father and stepmother in Detroit, the home of Motown. We started dating in our senior year of high school, and he shared the Motown sound with me at the end of each summer when he returned from Detroit.

I've always been an embarrassed and clumsy dancer, but alcohol helped me at the Jacksons' party. Several couples at a time were able to squeeze in and dance on the ten-by-twelve living room floor. I did the waltz, cha-cha, and jitterbug in my junior high years in Illinois when my parents sent me to ballroom dancing classes at a boys' academy. I did the twist at my friend Fifi's house there in Wheaton when I was in high school. And I'd sort of faked it at school dances after games at Oshkosh High. I remember going out on the floor with Bill, the first boy I ever dated, because it seemed like a slow dance was being played, and then being embarrassed when the tempo picked up.

This night, in the Jacksons' trailer, Rufus touched my shoulder and said, "Want to dance?"

I couldn't very well say no. He proceeded to dance with me up close. Luckily, I was loose from drinking beer by this time, so I survived it despite my embarrassment.

The Jacksons' party was mostly for college students and the Jacksons' friends from their hometown, so Maybelle and Joseph Henry hadn't been invited. Maybelle asked me to come visit the next day at their mobile home which was parked across the center driveway behind Buddy. the mobile home. Their mobile home was ten feet longer than ours, as needed for the couple and their two children and because Maybelle did women's hair in their home.

Maybelle and Joseph Henry were Geechee Gullah, from an area near Brunswick, Georgia, that for a long time was largely separate from other Georgia communities.

"I'm the first Geechee you met, I can tell," Maybelle said as we sat at their kitchen table. "Geechee don't take no mess. You don't want to make us mad. One day, this ol' dog come in the yard barking, and I got my gun and shot 'im."

Her little girl, Florine, was playing with a doll nearby as she said this. Her son was trying to open a box, and she told him, "Junior, I told you! Don't be fooling with that. You bad!"

I couldn't see what Junior was fooling with, but I was impressed with Maybelle's spirit.

The Jackson's trailer faced our back door. Out our front door, I could see David Carswell's trailer. Coming from his windows — or walls — I could hear the music of Isaac Hayes, Pharoah Sanders (an avant-garde jazz musician), and, later, James Taylor who sang, "You've Got a Friend." David introduced me to these artists (I was impressed by the jazz of Pharoah Sanders) and also shared a beer from Florida that had pineapple and coconut flavoring.

David loved to talk, and laugh, and he almost aways wore a friendly smile.

"Our daddy works at the country club in Macon. Worked there at least twenty years," David explained while we were standing out in the yard. "Now we have a club on Poplar Street in Macon, Peyton Place. Named it after my brother Peyton. He's married. I'm in graduate school and my girlfriend Miriam comes down here weekends. She work at Armstrong in Macon, in the office."

I met Miriam later, a gracious young woman with a beautiful medium-length afro. David's other brother, Harold or "Blake," showed up occasionally. He looked like David but with a hard edge and fewer smiles. He was involved in the black power movement.

In this small trailer park on the edge of town, I wasn't just exposed to people from various cultures, I was getting to know them as friends and neighbors.

11.

"We Shall Overcome"

S OON AFTER classes began, the college's Cooperative Extension
Program hosted a dinner at Camp John Hope, a youth camp
located a few miles out in the country. My friend and agriculture
researcher Ron Abe explained to me that Georgia had two
Cooperative Extension Services serving Georgia's counties. One,
with one of its local offices in Fort Valley, served farmers in Peach
County and reported directly to the University of Georgia. The other,
the Fort Valley State Cooperative Extension, also reported to UGA,
and it sent agents out to assist black farmers both in the local area
and all over Georgia. The two extensions exist separately even today,
though the FVSU Cooperative Extension now assists many small
farmers, not only blacks.

Ron, Scott, and I rode out together to the camp. By this time,
Ron had gotten his own mobile home set up on the other side of
Dr. Stallworth's house. Dr. Stallworth was one of Ron's agriculture
colleagues. Scott also had moved out of Stokey's apartments. Now
he lived in a house in a black neighborhood behind the college. The
house belonged to Clinton and Virginia Dixon, who were away
at school in Oklahoma, and it was being managed by Dr. Myland
Brown. Later in the year, Dr. Brown put Scott out. I didn't know
why. I thought maybe he didn't approve of the cats. At that time, the
Dixons had not returned from Oklahoma.

Ron pulled into my driveway first, so I got in the front seat. He
went around the campus to Scott's place, and Scott got in the back
seat. Then we headed out Carver Drive and out of town towards
Camp John Hope.

"This is way out in the country," observed Scott. "And it's hot."

"Hilo hot, too," said Ron, referring to the city where he grew up in Hawaii.

"It doesn't get hot very often where I'm from," I said. "And we're not ready for it when it does. I remember sweating on my pillowcase when I was trying to sleep."

We arrived and went up a dirt drive on a slight hill to the dining hall. The camp's set up with its main buildings and surrounding cottages reminded me a lot of Camp Alpine, the Lutheran camp I went to as a child back in Illinois. When the three of us entered the dining hall, I looked up and saw high ceilings. Tables were arranged in a large rectangle, and our dinners were served to us as they had been at the beginning of the year dinner in Bishop Hall.

The Cooperative Extension Program managed Camp John Hope since it was part of the agriculture division. Dr. Cozy Ellison, head of agriculture, was Ron's and Dr. Stallworth's boss. He would have sponsored the dinner and program.

Years later, Dr. Donnie Bellamy, a history professor at the college, explained to me the story behind our agriculture program. In 1947, Georgia's Board of Regents and the Georgia General Assembly moved the 1890 land grant designation from Savannah State College, the black college near the coast, to Fort Valley State, and some federal funding came with the move. Since Savanna State is near a seaport and we are in the middle of farm country, it made sense. Unfortunately, and unfairly, Georgia refused to give FVSC the federally stipulated percentage of land grant research funding from the federal government until around 2010. Almost all of every federal dollar Georgia received went to the predominantly white 1860 land grant institution, the University of Georgia. (UGA received its designation in 1872.)

Since 1947, the land grant mission has helped determine the role of Fort Valley State College, now University. The law not only states that the 1890 institutions should further agriculture research and education. It also designates their special academic mission: to educate those who are under-represented at other institutions, such as African Americans in the case of FVSC, and people with low incomes. The land grant mission specifically includes teaching and fostering the liberal arts. I didn't understand the Land Grant mission or know about the underfunding at the time.

I did enjoy the dinner. We had turkey, cornbread stuffing (which was new to me), and turnip greens, with the vinegar sauce in the little clear bottles containing the green peppers. I disliked the white bread stuffing people up north ate at Thanksgiving. My mother didn't like it either, but she prepared it since it was traditional for stuffing the turkey. We also had it at my aunt's house in Ohio the few times we went there for Thanksgiving. But this Georgia cornbread stuffing had some turkey flavor, increased by the gravy, and a mellow taste. I really liked it, and I have been making it myself ever since.

But before we ate, and after the prayer, we sang two songs together, "Lift Every Voice and Sing," the Negro national anthem, and "We Shall Overcome." We stood for "Lift Every Voice and Sing." I had to read the lyrics from the program, but most people in the room knew it by heart. We continued standing for "We Shall Overcome," and we held hands and swayed as we sang. I remembered learning about the civil rights movement from television and in school, and I knew that the recently assassinated Dr. Martin Luther King, Jr., and his followers sang the song. Now, the experience of singing that iconic song with black Americans who were my fellow citizens, literally made my skin tingle. I didn't feel like an outsider at that moment. I felt like a member of this large family.

12.

"Ha-ve some?"

RETURNING TO our office from my eleven o'clock class the next week, I found Mrs. Cook, Mrs. Adams, Mrs. Powell, and Mrs. Malone sitting down and ready to eat their lunches. Mrs. Malone produced hers from her desk.

"Ha-ve some?" she offered rather loudly, putting the emphasis on the second syllable.

"No thanks," mumbled the others, as if they had answered this question before.

I looked at Mrs. Cook, who sneaked a smile back at me.

Mrs. Powell and Mrs. Adams didn't even bother to look up.

Mrs. Malone seemed almost grandmotherly to me, not intellectual at all. She was Reverend Malone's second wife and did not have any children of her own. She called him "the Reverend." She and Miss Douglas seemed to be close friends, but I couldn't understand the basis of their friendship. Miss Douglas, very intelligent and up on her field, made a direct contrast with Mrs. Malone, with her old-fashioned way of speaking, and her reliance on high school instructors' manuals. I didn't understand then that there is more to friendship than appreciating each other's intelligence, mutual support being one of those things.

When it came to Mrs. Malone's daily invitation to share her lunch, I guessed that was an example of the southern hospitality I had heard about. I didn't experience southern hospitality all that much, except in our trailer park among our neighbors. I wasn't invited to more than one home outside of the park in my first few years in the South though I often heard people say, "Come see us, hear?"

I did hear the voice of southern hospitality in the voice of Mrs. Ethel Phelps, the college's telephone receptionist. When you telephoned Fort Valley State College, she answered every time in her melodious soprano voice with, "Hell-o-oo! May I help you?"

After lunch, it was time for me to teach my next class, English 321, the first part of Survey of British Literature. I did not use an instructor's manual. I did try to get this class off to a good start and show my enthusiasm for the classic works we were to cover. Miss Douglas assigned the survey courses to me because I'd had several graduate and undergraduate classes in British literature. And she chose the handbook we were supposed to use with the surveys, William Flint Thrall and Addison Hibbard's *A Handbook to Literature*, which became in later editions Thrall, Hibbard and Holman's *A Handbook to Literature*. In my college classes, I tried hard to learn the literary devices and characteristics of the literature of different periods. Now, in one book, I found practically everything I'd learned.

Every class day, I entered room 211 and looked around at the English majors sitting in the old metal and wood desks. Almost all of them were young women, and since they were juniors, all only about two years younger than me.

Remembering the southern way, I'd greet them, "Good morning! How are you doing today?"

"Fine, thank you," they'd say with a notable lack of enthusiasm.

In their main text, *The Literature of England*, we read *Beowulf* in a modern translation and were working on *Sir Gawain and the Green Knight*, also in a modern translation. Today, I tried to explain that Middle English was spoken differently—in different dialects—in different parts of England, and that our next readings, from Geoffrey Chaucer's *Canterbury Tales*, were going to be in a dialect closer to ours, so the text was not in a modern translation in their book.

"We'll learn how to pronounce the Middle English words, and we'll practice," I said. "The beginning of the poem—the 'Prologue,' is famous. It starts like this, 'Whan that Aprille with his shoures soote/The droughte of Marche hath perced to the roote—'"

Some of the young ladies were talking in low voices to each other, but when I came out with those strange sounding words, they looked up and laughed.

"Your book explains how to pronounce the words, and there are lots of footnotes to explain words you may not recognize," I encouraged them, ignoring the snickers. But they did not look like they thought they were going to enjoy this.

"When I was in college," I said, "I practiced with a recording by Helga Kokeritz. If I can find a record player, I'll play it for you so you can try to imitate the pronunciations."

They just looked at me.

I'd been trying to get discussions going without much luck. Now I was trying to get them involved by asking questions like, "What do you think makes Beowulf a hero?"

These young ladies, within a year of going out to be teachers themselves, probably would get married in the near future and had never had a young, white, female teacher from the North before. Patricia, whose father was in the Army at Fort Benning, chatted with me sometimes. But we talked in the office or after class, not as a part of the class dynamics.

Eventually, to help the English majors, I developed key concepts for the class with related images, such as the Golden Chain of Being that describes the Renaissance concept of hierarchy with God at the top, then the angels, then the ruler, with the common man and animals at the bottom. I hoped they would associate the literature they were reading with the historical time periods the literature came from.

After the not-so-successful British Literature class, I returned to the office to get ready for Freshman Composition, or English 101.

"I wish I could get the English majors interested in the literature," I said to JC, who was in the office when I got back.

"Assign them to teach parts of it. Then they'll do the reading. Sure will!" he suggested.

"Maybe," I said. "I don't know if there's time for me to teach what's important and do that, too."

If most of my English majors were non-committal and unengaged, JC with his curly hair and frequent smiles certainly was the opposite. He told me he'd been in the Army, he had a house in Atlanta even though he taught full time in Fort Valley, and he traveled with the debate team, which he coached. His given name really was JC. It didn't stand for anything. He managed to be both cheerful and fatalistic about our obstacles as English instructors, all at the same time. I can still picture him lifting the pitch of his voice to complain about something, then smiling and shaking his head.

"Sure do!" he'd say about the behavior of the students or whatever colleagues we were discussing. Later, JC married Wilhemena, a young woman from the local area, and he moved to Fort Valley to raise his family. He coached debate for years and even ran a radio station and started a videography business with his son, Jarrett.

It was five years since my time as a student in English composition class back at Oshkosh State, and I didn't remember much about it. Now, at Fort Valley State College, our book for Freshman English contributed to the students' learning and to mine, as well. *Staircase to Writing and Reading*, written by Alan Casty and Donald Tighe, did not teach the process method for writing that has found favor since the nineteen-eighties and nineties. But it did help the students practice and understand the elements of an essay and how they are related logically to the main argument of a paper. It also had a section on argumentation and logic. I'm not so sure about the students, but I referred back to the elements laid out in this text many times as the years went by.

At twenty-three, I thought of myself as fully adult and I thought of all my students, even my freshmen, as adults. I was less conscious that my students were close in age to me. I met a wide cross section of Fort Valley State College students while teaching beginning freshmen. I taught nearly a hundred students a year in these classes. I always asked them to introduce themselves and say where they were from, and I formed a mental picture of many towns and cities in Georgia this way. Teresa, from Tifton, had beautiful curly hair and a dimpled smile and always did her work. Lavonne, like many students who came from the City of Fort Valley where the college was located, was well-mannered, friendly, and serious. Alfreda, who was from Perry, sticks in my mind. She wrote that her mother made her wear a raincoat, but when she was away from the house, she said, "I took off my raincoat and went to my destiny."

I taught science majors, business majors, ROTC cadets (though they were not officially connected to enlistment in officer training through the college program yet) and athletes, male and female, from all the sports. I'll never forget seeing my student, Cadet Isaac Lightfoot, marching in the Homecoming parade. He was very tall, very big, and appeared to have very big and heavy, not light, feet.

Many of my students made a lot of errors in what I called standard English. (I think now that it's better to refer to it as business English.) Although I was strict in grading, I valued intelligence and gave weight to a good argument, good support, and originality over grammar. My linguistics class at Wisconsin had not been my best subject. I got a B, which was the lowest acceptable grade in graduate school. But I did learn about different dialects in different geographical areas of the US, and I learned that language evolves rather than, as the French preferred to think, remaining static with clear divisions between right and wrong. Discussion about Ebonics, led by Geneva Smitherman, had just begun at the time I came to FVSC.

In my freshman English classes, the students were attentive and alive. The young men were funny, often aiming for a reaction when they spoke, and when the young women reacted with giggles to their male counterparts, they were cute. I had no preparation for teaching, only my own education, and in all of my classes, I simply got down to business and shared my knowledge and what was in their texts. I had a purpose to focus on while Mike was away at Fort Benning.

13.

"The Other America"

MIKE WAS NOT ABLE to take leave the weekend I received an invitation from Dr. Constance Palms to come to her house for tea. Dr. Palms, one of Miss Douglas's friends, told me Gladys Porter, a sociology instructor, would be coming over too. Miss Porter picked me up and, as they say in Georgia, "carried" me to Dr. Palms' house on Vineville, a street near Five Points, the main intersection in town. The little frame house had a porch and was very neat and well-furnished inside.

"This dining-room table and chairs and the tea set were my mother's," Dr. Palms said. "Do you take sugar?"

I was glad she asked. Most southerners seemed to assume that people take sugar in iced tea (they call it "sweet tea"), hot tea, and coffee. At least that's what my limited social opportunities had indicated so far.

"No, thank you," I said. (I decided not to mention like I usually did that my parents didn't use sugar in tea or coffee.) "Thank you for inviting me! Most of the faculty members I've met so far are either in the English Department or they are new faculty, like I am."

"My office is in Peabody, and Constance is in Hubbard Education," Miss Porter said. "We all see each other at faculty meetings, Founders Day, and the Christmas tree lighting. The rest of the time we tend to stay in our little areas."

"I understand this is your first teaching job," said Dr. Palms.

"Yes, unless you count teaching Sunday School," I answered, trying for some modest humor. "I thought about teaching high school at

one time, but I wanted to be a college professor like my dad. Anyway,
I'm the oldest child in my family, but I'm not good at making kids
behave. The preacher's kid in the Sunday School class I taught always
gave me a hard time. College students behave like adults, and I enjoy
teaching my classes and talking to them after class. Sometimes they
joke around a little, but that's OK."

"What street is your house on?" I went on, trying to make
conversation.

"This is Vineville," Dr. Palms said, "and that's what the black
neighborhood behind me is called. We have several black neighborhoods in Fort Valley, not just the ones around the college campus."

I heard later about houses in Vineville that sold liquor illegally.
They were called shot houses because people could buy drinks by
the shot. Shot houses exist in Fort Valley to this day.

"Going to work," I observed, "I pass a neighborhood across the
street from the campus where old trailers are mixed in with houses."

Miss Porter said, "That is Gano. If you turn and go across the
tracks heading out of town on highway 96, you'll go past another
black neighborhood called Griffinline."

After a while, I learned that more neighborhoods became integrated every year (meaning somebody black bought a house in a
white neighborhood) and then turned largely black. That's what
happened around my Uncle Happy's house in Toledo. I credit him
because he and his family stayed put in the midst of that change.

"Some of our college instructors and public school teachers live
on the streets in back of the campus, behind the College Inn," Dr.
Palms added as she offered me a slice of pound cake.

I'll never forget the kindness of Dr. Palms and Miss Porter to
have me over and share some knowledge of the city and the college
with me.

Saturday at suppertime, Ron and Scott planned to go to the nearby
city of Macon to eat and have some beer, and they asked me to come
along. We went to Lum's on Pio Nono where the specialty was hot
dogs and where a huge refrigerator held beer from all over the world.

In Wisconsin, where beer was cheap due to not being taxed, I didn't care for beer. Now in Georgia, where it was expensive, I started to enjoy some brews. I wasn't so sure about the Florida beer David shared with me at Stallworth's Trailer Park, though.

"I drink mostly beer," Ron said. "This place have Hawaii and Japan beer."

"Beer is OK," said Scott. "But Tennessee makes bourbon and whiskey. I think moonshine comes from Georgia."

"I think a lot of churches here are against drinking, like the Free Church and Bible Church were in Wheaton where I grew up," I said. "Oshkosh is the opposite. We moved there when I was sixteen. There's a tavern on practically every corner. People bring their kids in on Fridays for fish fries. The perch is really good!"

"That lake fish," Ron said. "I like ocean fish."

He opened another bottle of beer and poured it in his glass.

"We used to go north to my grandparents' cabin in Minnesota every year, and I can tell you, there's nothing like fresh pan fish—perch, blue gill, and sunfish," I argued.

I had been to the ocean only once on a family vacation. I loved Northern lakes.

"We're getting some new faculty in CEAP," Scott said. "Are you getting any new instructors?"

"We just got Peter Dolce," I said. "He doesn't say much, but I think he's from New York or Philadelphia, one of those Northeastern states."

"We get new researchers, but not more instructors," Ron said. "The farmers need help."

When Ron, Scott, and I drove out to look at the countryside earlier that week, we saw houses that black families lived in, usually on the property of white farmers who had large, white farmhouses. The black tenant farmers or farm hands and their families lived in houses that looked as if they had never been painted. I learned that many of them had to go to a well every day to pump their water, and they used outhouses. My Great Aunt Mert's house in central Ohio had an outhouse, but I figured that was just because she and her house were old. We had an outhouse and pump at my grandparents' cottage, but that was like camping by the lake. It didn't seem right for families with children to live like that in Georgia now.

As if he knew what I had been thinking about, Ron said, "Doc Stallworth say some of the black children living on those farms we saw don't go to school."

"In my American cultural history class, we read a book called *The Other America*," I said, remembering what these houses in the country reminded me of. "It had pictures of houses in the rural South a lot like the ones we saw. I guess it's taking a long time to get over the poverty they had from erosion and the boll weevil and maybe from the Civil War."

"We do have a lot of small farms in Tennessee," Scott admitted as we were sitting there eating our hot dogs. "And some of those little wood houses in the hills aren't fancy. But I think people own their own places even if they're not that well off."

In addition to the people living in poor situations in Georgia, I saw many skinny, mangy dogs on my side of town. I believed in stopping to help any animal I saw in need, but in Georgia I felt too overwhelmed.

Worried our cats could be attacked by the stray dogs, I put a pen in the yard in front of our mobile home. When they were outside, Pokey and Fu wore harnesses and were on leashes hooked to a metal stake in the middle of the protective pen.

I told Mike about the pen and leashes and the houses out in the country when he called.

"Oh, yeah?" he said. "Georgia's a strange place. Guess what? I did my first jump! I'm officially a paratrooper, and you're not, so you're a 'leg.' Ranger training is next—I'll tell you about it."

We hung up, and I focused back on where I was and on my work.

14.

Scoping

I T WAS TIME for the Scope Chart interviews at the college. Even though FVSC faculty had been told they weren't supposed to serve *in loco parentis* anymore, the Scope Chart requirement was still in place during my first year. With my desk in the middle of the room surrounded by other English faculty, I was to interview students assigned to me on their Scope Chart progress in spite of the lack of privacy. As an English instructor, I taught a lot of freshmen, so it was freshmen I was assigned to advise.

The Scope Chart was created in 1940, and from then until around 1969, the college faculty assisted the students in "achieving the objectives the college deems essential to a well-rounded personality." As advisor, I was the "Scoper," and the students were the "Scopees." I had to meet with the freshmen assigned to me at least two times each during the school year and assign points each quarter so they could earn the total number required for graduation. Of course, to graduate, the students also had to meet all the academic requirements including a satisfactory grade point average and completion of their required courses and number of hours.

A simplified version of the Scope Chart was posted on the wall in our combined office, and individual freshmen received their own charts in the form of booklets to be filled in during conferences and kept by the advisor to be passed on to the student's new advisor at the end of each school year. I already had the Survey of British Literature class containing about twenty students, another upper division literature class with about ten students, and three freshman and sophomore classes with about thirty students each. My Scopees gave me five more students to think about.

On my first day as a Scope advisor, I had two appointments, with freshman students I'll call Luther and Barbara Ann. Barbara Ann came in first, peering into the large room to find me. Mr. McGhee and Mrs. Powell were working at their desks, but they remained quiet so as not to distract us. I moved some of my books and papers on my desk to make room.

"Hi, I'm Mrs. Mitchell. Are you Barbara Ann Jenkins?"

"Yes, Ma'am."

"You can sit here. We've got to go through this booklet to see where you are at the present time. You'll keep this booklet the whole time you are in college. I'll turn it in when the year's up, and it will be passed on to your new advisor next year. I'm just going to ask you the questions that are in the book."

I didn't have to do anything remotely similar to this in college or even high school. At Oshkosh State College, we had advisors based on our majors, but we really only discussed what classes to take when we went to see them. I do remember my advisor, an older professor, leaning back and explaining to me that he was a conservative in the English sense — more of a royalist. He did not seem to be guiding or disciplining me, just being conversational.

I felt a little awkward being a Scope Chart advisor, but I was already getting used to playing the role of instructor.

Barbara Ann was a very polite young woman, wearing a blue skirt that was a little below her knees (not the mini-skirt some had started wearing to class). She had medium-length hair that had been straightened and put into waves. She sat in the chair beside my desk, smelling a little like a macaroon. It took me a minute to figure out that she used coconut oil in her hair. I opened her Scope Chart booklet with its pages and pages of questions and possible points. Some of them depended on the student's word about personal habits and hygiene. It embarrassed me to talk about these, even with a female who was younger than me.

"I'm supposed to ask whether you keep up with good health prac-
tices, practice cleanliness, and refrain from excessive smoking, do
not consume alcoholic beverages or narcotics and do not engage in
illicit sex," I told her.

In my embarrassment and haste to get through this part, I merged
three main points with their five sub-points in my question.

The Scope Chart Objective I, Health, contained fourteen
subpoints under A, four subpoints under B, and ten sub-points
under C. Many of the sub-points had their own subpoints. (The
other objectives included: II. Earning a Living, III. Citizenship, IV.
Utilizing and Controlling the Natural Environment for Individual
and Social Needs, V. Communication (Receiving and Transmitting
Ideas), VI. Expressing Athletic Impulses, VII. Utilizing Education
as a Means of Acquiring and Transmitting the Social Heritage and
as an Agency for Conserving and Improving Human and Material
Resources, and VIII. The Good Life.) Each objective encompassed
many sub-points and sub-sub-points.

"Yes Ma'am," Barbara Ann responded, and I gave her full points
for Health.

It was easier when I could ask her which sports or other activities she had participated in and, later, which clubs she had been a
member of or an officer in. Apparently, she was not expected to get
full points in every area because, for one thing, she had four years to
acquire all the needed points. For another thing, she could get more
points in areas she was especially interested in, in case she got fewer
points in things she was not interested in. Barbara Ann had not been
an officer in anything yet, but she did sing in the choir, for example.

I suspected that some other advisors, like Mrs. Malone, acted
like parents when they asked the students these questions. I always
wanted to treat my students as equal adults, although I did lecture
them if I thought they had done something that really was not
correct. Being answered with "Yes, Ma'am," still made me uncomfortable although I was getting used to it.

"You're doing great so far," I told Barbara Ann. "I'll see you next quarter, and you can come by and see me before that if you have any questions or if you need to talk."

Luther more-or-less loomed in the doorway before he entered the office. He was a second year freshman. He had not passed enough classes the previous year to be considered a sophomore, so he and his Scope Chart came to me this year even though he was a little older. Besides being tall, he was built like an athlete. Luther wore starched and pressed blue jeans with the crease down the front, brown dress boots, and a gray and blue double-knit sweater, long sleeved, with a collar and a band at the hip so it fit well without being tucked in—not the team shirt and hat we'd see today. I figured he'd do well on the questions about athletics and team or group involvement.

"Do you show loyalty to the college?" I asked him, reading from the booklet, "by carrying on the following: speaking about your teachers and fellow students in complimentary terms away from the school and attempting to solve your problems through the proper channels?"

"Ah, yes ma'am. But at home I don't talk about school. My friends ain't in college, and I don't want to act like I'm so much."

The Scope Chart with its eight objectives and multiple subpoints didn't directly address this issue. But I saw the problem he faced.

"My dad went to college," I said, "but he was good at talking with my uncles on my mother's side who didn't go. So, I know what you mean."

Luther looked like he accepted this expression of my own experience.

"I got to get my grade point up so I can pledge," he offered. "Some of the questions in here is about leadership and like that."

"Well," I suggested, "that would be good. But getting good grades also is important because it means you are learning, and what you learn, along with the grades, will help you get a good job, maybe in a company, since you're a business major."

In fact, I had no idea what these African American students in the South, especially the average ones, would face when they finished college and looked for a position in the workforce.

Luther looked relieved when we got through all the questions, and I'm sure I looked relieved, too. He thanked me, got up from the chair by my desk, unfolding his six-foot-plus frame, and exited the big office.

Overall, the Scope Chart seemed odd, though well-intentioned. I felt that having the students talk about life with an instructor was a good thing, or it could be.

15.

Mrs. Lemon and Peewee

I STILL COULDN'T DRIVE and I didn't have a car, but I could walk from my office in the Academic Building to nearby black businesses. The Shrimp Boat, one street over from the back of the campus, sold fried fish and shrimp that I liked. That's when I started the habit of eating tartar sauce with my fried shrimp. I had lunch sometimes at the College Inn, a small restaurant directly behind the campus and not far at all from my office. JC told me it was owned by Mr. and Mrs. Lemon.

"Miss Leola's friendly," he said, "but she don't take any foolishness."

The first time I came into the College Inn and looked around, I saw a counter and a few tables and chairs. Behind the counter I saw a small older lady who wore an apron and appeared to be in charge. That was Mrs. Lemon.

I looked at the posted menu and chose a chicken sandwich, potatoes, and a milk to drink.

"I'd like to get a chicken sandwich and potatoes—"

"Ice potatoes?" Mrs. Lemon asked.

"Uh, french fries?" I responded. "And I want milk to drink—"

"White milk?" Mrs. Lemon asked.

I wondered what other kind there was, but I said, "Yes."

I learned that ice potatoes are actually Irish—that is, not sweet—potatoes. Not that many people ordered milk at the College Inn, but it was more likely to be chocolate if they did. And the chicken sandwich was not what I expected. It was a quarter of a fried chicken between two slices of white bread. I was thinking of chicken salad or sliced chicken meat. If I had gotten a carbonated drink, no matter what kind, it would have been a "Co-cola."

Leaving the College Inn, I crossed the street and headed back to The Yard. Maybe I'll check my mail, I thought, so I went between the Academic Building and Bywaters and turned left. As I approached the main sidewalk, I saw a short, thin man I'd noticed before in the student center. He had wavy hair, a little longer than typical.

"How're you doin' Peewee?" a student called to him.

"Fine," Peewee answered. "How you doin' Bobby?"

As I approached, Peewee pulled a deck of cards from his pants pocket and asked Bobby to pick one.

"Not today, man," Bobby said. "I'm wanting to see what you got. Any bracelets? My girlfriend, she wants one."

Peewee pulled some envelopes from his bag and let Bobby look.

"May I see?" I asked, walking up closer. Peewee opened some of the envelopes and held up beaded bracelets. Some beads were oblong and dark, and others were red, yellow, turquoise, and white.

"Do you make earrings?" I asked. "I've been making earrings with beads and wire. And do you have any necklaces?"

"I been making them," he said. "I'll bring some. Where you at?"

"I'm Anna Mitchell, and I'm in the English Department."

"He's Peewee Tukes," Bobby said. "He's a magician and he makes jewelry."

The next week, I saw Peewee's table in the student center. And I bought a necklace. It had a silver-colored chain punctuated by groupings of dark and turquoise-colored beads and a pendant cut out of silver-colored metal in the shape of a flying eagle. Next to me at the table, a teen-aged girl looked at the brass bangles, then picked out a bracelet made from a spoon near a display of small brass earrings. These were cut in the shape of Africa. Before I left the table, I couldn't resist buying one of Peewee's bags of peanuts. I'd been talked into buying boiled peanuts earlier, and I hated them. For me, a northerner, roasted peanuts were a treat.

Years later, Sam Henderson, a Fort Valley student who knew and talked to Peewee on campus in the eighties, shared with me things Peewee told him and his friends.

According to Sam, Peewee would say, "What's black is white and what's white is black," and that meant the world would tell college-educated black men to work for others and build their legacy, but they could build their own legacies. Peewee also would say, "I've seen so many of you young boys come to Fort Valley State College and go on to get 'good' jobs, but I have not seen any of you use your education to create a payroll for those like you that can't get a college degree."

Peewee had his own little business selling peanuts and making and selling jewelry, maybe the best he could do with his fragile body and in this small southern town. But he dreamed of black men who could create and grow larger businesses, employing and helping other black people.

According to Henderson, Peewee knew people looked at him and saw a suffering man, but he said, "I chose the life I live. I am content. I have a roof over my head, and I make enough money to feed myself."

More recently Mr. Herbert the jeweler said about Peewee that he had used some of the jeweler's tools to cut out pendants and earrings. Peewee Tukes had such a talent, Herbert said, that he could make his way in New York City.

16.

White Merchants and a Black Ceremony

THE STORE OWNERS Dennis Herbert and his wife Peggy made me feel welcome as did a few other white business owners. But not all did.

The tellers at the Bank of Fort Valley were the worst.

Once I had a paycheck, I needed a bank account, so I set one up at that bank which was located on the main thoroughfare. I planned to bring my paychecks there each month to be deposited. I felt a little uncomfortable on my first visit, but I didn't dwell on it since everything was new to me.

The next time I walked into their lobby, I realized the all white staff stopped what they were doing and looked across the room at me when I entered. I went over to a high table in the middle of the room to write out my deposit slip, then glanced back up at the tellers behind the counter. They continued to stare down at me. No smiles.

As I stepped up to the raised service counter, suddenly I understood. I was the white girl working at the colored school, they'd apparently heard. And I was a Yankee, to boot. I put my check back in my purse and went back out to where Scott was waiting for me.

"I don't think those people are very nice," I told him. "I don't want that to be my bank."

"You can close your account," he said.

So, I braved the stares a second time, went back in, withdrew what money I had, and closed the account.

I changed to Citizens Bank farther down the street, where I was treated in a decent, businesslike way. In fact, they were friendly and recognized me pleasantly every time I came in. They have served me well ever since. They even gave me a loan in 1979 so I could pay for an airline ticket to go to Ohio and defend my dissertation. In recent years, the name of Citizens Bank has been changed to Synovus, and the tellers still say, "Hi, Miss Anna!"

I shopped for food at the A&P, the same grocery chain my mother patronized when I was growing up. I got the same French dressing and mayonnaise and Eight O'clock Coffee. One of the cashiers exhibited the southern hospitality I had heard about, speaking kindly to me and asking how I was doing. As I interacted with this lady and with a lady at the Citizens Bank (I seem to remember that they were sisters), and a few others, like Mrs. Hester who was the wife of a convenience store owner, I came to what I thought was a fair conclusion. Every day, these women wore dresses, they seemed to have their hair done by beauticians, and they had make-up on. They were a lot more dressed up than I was and even more dressed up than the mothers of my friends back in Oshkosh, who, in turn, were more dressed up than my own mother. I had heard the tag, "Southern Belle." These ladies had to go out and work to help support their families unlike my mom and many of my friends' moms in the Midwest. At the same time, they still had to be gracious and lovely southern belles. They did seem a bit tired.

I didn't want to be a southern belle, but I did want outfits to wear to work that looked a little trendy and were sufficiently professional. Both Par-San and Khoury's Women's Wear in downtown Fort Valley seemed to have good skirts, tops, and even matching pants and tops for me to wear to work. I thought Khoury's was more up to date. I prowled the row of pants outfits, looking for slacks, maybe even bell bottoms, but with matching tops so I'd look appropriate for a working woman and college instructor. Then the owner Lorraine Khoury and I began to talk. (Like my mother, I like to chat with strangers.)

"How do you like Fort Valley?" she asked. She wasn't fazed to hear that I had a job at the black college.

"I'm still getting acquainted with everything," I told her. "I like this pants suit, it's denim, but I think I can wear it to teach in since it's a complete outfit. I want to buy this."

Lorraine wore a skirt and top and had her short dark blonde hair in a simple style, not curled and hair-sprayed like some other Fort Valley women. She appeared to be close to my age. Later on, when I finally got my ears pierced, I created earrings from copper wire and beads of light blue stone, red coral, white quartz, and multicolored red, white, blue, and brown ceramic. Lorraine offered to sell them on commission at the store, and she put a little revolving rack on the counter for them. That was fun, although I don't recall selling very many.

I didn't assume the worst of all white folks in Fort Valley because I realized their upbringing was probably quite different from mine, and some, at least, were trying to adjust to change, like Buddy Smisson at the Gulf Station.

We simply had few black citizens in the towns where I grew up, so I couldn't guarantee Wheaton or Oshkosh would have been much freer of prejudice than southern towns if more African Americans lived there. I just knew my own parents had taught us to respect other people. In the City of Fort Valley, even though I went to white banks, grocery stores, clothing stores, and hardware stores, I didn't get to know any townspeople socially, so I wasn't sure what they thought. A few of the merchants spoke to me in a friendly, sociable way, but more of them didn't.

Very little of my time was spent in the stores of Fort Valley. Mostly, I continued my immersion in the traditions of Fort Valley State College. A big one was about to take place.

"Do you have your academic attire?" Miss Douglas asked one day as I stood in her office.

"No," I admitted, "I didn't attend the commencement for my master's. We were getting ready to move to Georgia."

"You must go down to the bookstore and order a rental. You need the gown, the hood, and the cap. You'll need them in the spring for graduation, too, but we wear our regalia every year for Founders Day. That will be in a few weeks."

On Founders Day, the group of men who came together to create a school for blacks in Fort Valley as well as two of the first leaders of the school are honored. Dr. Donnie Bellamy explains in *Light in the Valley: A Pictorial History of Fort Valley State College Since 1895* that the event called Founders Day began in 1940 to remember Henry A. Hunt and later, after she passed, Florence Johnson Hunt. I had noticed a photograph of Henry A. Hunt on the wall of St. Luke's Parish Hall when I attended that church across the street from the Carnegie Building. I learned that Hunt, who focused on industrial education, came from Hancock County, graduated from Atlanta University, and taught in grammar schools and at Johnson C. Smith University, before coming to Fort Valley High and Industrial in 1904 as its second principal.

Today, another educator in Georgia also is honored on Fort Valley State's annual Founders Day. Before Fort Valley became a state school and focused on agriculture, a black agricultural college was in Forsyth. William Hubbard was the founder of The State Teachers and Agricultural College of Forsyth. That college closed, and beginning in 1940, Fort Valley State College also celebrated Hubbard Day. (We always thought that the colleges had merged, but that is not exactly what happened.) Bellamy writes, "During the presidency of Waldo W. E. Blanchet, the two 'Founder's' Days, one to remember the Hunts and the other to remember William M. Hubbard were ended and one day continued...as 'Founders' Day.'"

Just as Miss Douglas had told me, the faculty, wearing their academic regalia, assembled more-or-less by rank over at the Miller Science Building on the big day. I wore my master's hood in Wisconsin colors over my robe for the first time. All around me stood fellow faculty members in their black robes wearing different colors of trim on their hoods. Some of the caps worn by those with EdDs or PhDs looked like flat berets instead of the mortarboards worn by those of us who only had master's degrees. Someone—a faculty or staff member—kept telling us to line up by rank, but it looked to me like the faculty members just kept on talking to each other. Finally, the music started, and we marched across into the Woodward Gymnasium following the president, the guest speaker, and other administrators. We listened to the featured speaker.

Then the roll call of the men who founded the college began. As it has since my first Founders' Day, the ceremony in the gymnasium always included a recitation of the names of these eighteen men, fifteen blacks (Henry Lowman, Peter Fann, James Isaac Miller, Thomas W. Williams, Thomas A. McAfee, John W. Davison, Gideon Virgil Barnett, Charlie H. Nixon, Charlie A. Anderson, Lee O'Neal, Alan Cooper, Alonzo N. Nixon, J.R. Jones, David Jones, DL Lawrence) and three whites, (Stephen Elisha Bassett, Francis W. Gano, and John Edward Hale) with a description of each man's race (black or white) and occupation.

After this part of the ceremony, we marched back up the campus, past the student center, Ohio Hall, the Hunt Library, and the Academic Building to the grave at the front of the campus where we sang the Alma Mater and other songs, including "Lift Every Voice and Sing," led by the college choir. I took note of all the proceedings. Little did I know that I would participate in this ceremony and see my fellow faculty members behave in about the same way forty-three more times. I left for graduate school for three years or it would have been forty-six.

I took part in more and more rituals and events at the college. I also read Mike's letters, composed my own, and thought about the constant changes occurring in my own life as Mike continued to be trained as a Second Lieutenant and to go to Vietnam.

17.

A Raven, a Lion, and a Car

———————————

MIKE CAME HOME for about a day after Ranger school, and then he flew to Fort Ord, California, to begin his officer training. When I had a break, I flew out to see him. The thought that he would be going to Vietnam when his training was finished hung over me. Still, the base was beautiful, and I was glad to spend a few days with him.

The first night, Mike was in one building in a set of barracks, and I stayed in a dormitory especially for wives and other family members. I slept in the narrow bed and got dressed in the morning following the regimen of an Army wife just as Mike was following the regimen of an officer in training.

In the morning, feeling happy and excited, I started across a broad grassy area in the middle of the base to find Mike. Suddenly I was dive-bombed by enormous black birds. I'm proud of not being the squeamish type, and I never scream, but I still hadn't gotten over the experience of watching Hitchcock's *The Birds*.

Luckily someone out there saw me and yelled, "Ravens! Your hair, they're after your hair!"

I snatched my long blondish hair, pulled it together, and stuffed it inside the neck of my navy-blue turtleneck.

Our experiences as a couple in California were mixed. It was good that we got to stay in a hostel for visiting wives and their husbands, and we were going to be able to travel off the base.

After I put my things in the room there, Mike said, "Come on out to the parking lot. I have something to show you."

I saw a new Volkswagen fastback with a shiny tan finish, complete with California license plates.

"This is our car," he told me.

He opened the door and we got inside.

"Now I really need to learn to drive and get my driver's license," I vowed.

It wasn't like I hadn't wanted to learn, but I'd missed out on drivers ed in high school when we moved after I turned sixteen, and my dad had been too busy working on his dissertation to teach me. Mom couldn't drive. She didn't learn until around 1972 when my little brother was in high school.

Now Mike was at the wheel of our new car, going up and down and around the sandy-colored hills on narrow roads in the mountainous area around Fort Ord going east from Monterey Bay. I wanted to see more of the Rockies. I'd been as far west as Colorado before, when I went to the Rampart Mountain Freedom School in the summer of 1965. There I saw mountainsides of rock and high meadows full of flowers. These northern California foothills were dry with fewer signs of vegetation.

We saw green hills and reddish rocks, and the sky was completely clear.

"These hills are beautiful," I said. Then, coming around a curve, we hit a beautiful mountain lion. I think we got out and looked at it to see if it was still alive. I can't remember. The vision of that beautiful lifeless body is what remains in my mind to this day. I know that grief and horror filled me as I looked at the large light brown animal lying beside the road. I love all animals, and especially cats. I would have been thrilled to see a live mountain lion up close. Knowing how I felt about animals, Mike tried to console me. But there was nothing we could do.

After that, we rode in silence for a while. Then I gradually tried small talk. We only had a short time together, so we had to make the best of it.

The evening ended at a restaurant on Fisherman's Wharf in Monterey where our table looked out over the water. I had a white fish covered with red Italian sauce. It was very good and something I wouldn't have thought of. I knew that our time together was almost over. The next day, I'd take a bus back to the airport and Mike would continue his training.

Our new tan Volkswagen Fastback was shipped back to Georgia by the Army when Mike's training in California was finished. His next assignment was to be Fort Bragg in North Carolina. He now had the prerequisites of being a paratrooper and a Ranger, and he had volunteered to be in the Special Forces, an elite unit who trained at Fort Bragg.

Ron also bought a VW fastback. His was light blue. Ron liked his car, but he felt guilty.

"I not getting any more cars not made in United States," he decided. "I want to support America."

I think that after World War II his family and other Japanese in Hilo and throughout Hawaii valued being loyal to the United States and wanted to show it.

Of the two Fort Valley State friends I hung out with, Scott and Ron, Scott was more like a buddy and a peer. He was my age. Ron, who had met Mike over at the Stallworth trailer park, tried to take on the role of helper and protector during Mike's absences. I accepted that although I thought of myself as independent. However, there was a limit to how independent I was while I couldn't drive.

I began taking driving lessons from Ron as soon as possible. After conquering the manual transmission and practicing with him for a while and learning from my brother Peter over the telephone how to parallel park, I was able to pass the driver's test.

During one of my driving lessons, Ron was in the front passenger seat and Scott rode in the back. We arrived in Macon and had to go up the hill on Pio Nono Avenue, a very steep hill with traffic lights. Even today, I tend to gun the gas when taking off up a hill if I'm driving a stick shift. I was much worse as a brand-new driver. At one traffic light I started going backwards before I got the clutch and gas-pedal synchronized. Scott gave a terrified shriek before we finally lurched forward. Ron remained calm, as always.

I didn't get around to changing the California license plate on the fastback, so people began assuming I was from California (except for those who still thought I was from Minnesota). I kept that license plate for quite a long time.

Mike returned from California and left the VW in Fort Valley with me when he reported to Fort Bragg.

18.

Exclusion and Inclusion

M IKE GOT A week's leave for Christmas and Fort Valley State College had winter breaks, so that year we went home to Oshkosh. Mike was dealing with a bad cold. For the first and only time, I stayed at his home instead of at my family's home. Mike's twin sisters, Jane and Jean, were home from college and in and out of the house during the holidays. At my family's house, my brother Peter was at home and still in high school. My sister was still at home, too. We opened gifts at both houses on Christmas, and the family celebrations went on as usual, but I felt a shadow over the festivities. The time for Mike to go to Vietnam was getting closer and closer.

After Christmas Day, Mike's cold got worse. The Mitchells' house, probably built in the 1920s, had an upstairs with dormers in the bedrooms, and Mike lay sick in the bed in one of those rooms with a serious cough and a fever. I found myself taking second place, standing helplessly out in the hall while Mrs. Mitchell (who, I admit, was a nurse) endeavored to take care of him. I had my own nurse complex and wanted to do that myself. Now that I'm the mother of sons, I realize his mother must have felt very emotional about his imminent departure and now about his being sick. I don't think I empathized with her at the time, being wrapped up in my own feelings.

Before New Year's Day, Mike recovered, and I went back to Georgia. Mike went back to Fort Bragg to complete the training to become a Green Beret. I was ambivalent, proud of him for being qualified to join the elite Special Forces but wanting to hold to the concept that we both were against the war. At one time, I thought, we had that in common with the hippies and the anti-war movement. This war used deadly force to try to achieve national objectives and, with the draft, applied coercion to its own young men. Faced with these contradictions between what I thought were our principles and what Mike seemed to be invested in now, I began to turn away from trying to justify myself or my husband to other people.

Winter quarter began at the college, and I continued teaching a variety of classes from the freshman to the junior level. There even were some seniors in my classes. I also started participating more in activities on campus outside the classroom. One show in the auditorium near the English office and one basketball game at the gym were especially memorable.

I went by myself to the show in the Academic Building auditorium, expecting to see a great performance by a troupe of female entertainers. The large auditorium had two sections, the lower one and the upper one. You could enter through the door in the middle or the one that led to the back of the auditorium. I went in the middle door and sat down on one of the wooden theater seats towards the back of the bottom section. Soon, women came out on stage singing and exhorting the audience to "Rise up!" Fort Valley State College regularly booked well-known black artists, so they probably were from a northern city, possibly New York.

Then I heard the women on the stage shout, "Whitey, whitey, get back!"

The players spoke to the audience, all of whom, except me, were black, and they shouted and sang about the struggle, directing some of their anger towards "honkeys" and "white whores." I felt small, sitting in my seat, wondering if anyone was looking at me or thinking about how I might feel, being called a "white whore." This show was my first glimpse of the black power movement or at least of black arts. I kept my mouth shut and took it all in as a learning experience. This culture was different from mine, and its people had gone through trials my people had not known.

In the 1968–69 season, Fort Valley State had the best basketball team in Wildcat history. It is hard to believe that just a few years earlier, the basketball games were played outdoors because Woodward Gymnasium had not yet been constructed. Now our team was in the process of becoming champions of the Southern Intercollegiate Athletic Conference (SIAC), a conference made up of black colleges and universities.

I've always loved basketball. My high school teams were good in their leagues, but the average player was thin, most all were white, and the guards were not particularly tall. At Wheaton Community High School, Coach Pfund's son John was one of my favorite players. He had an average size and build and played the guard position. Sonny Kee, a great multi-sport athlete and the only black player on Wheaton's varsity team at one point, played forward. His brother Dickie Kee, who played Junior Varsity basketball and then Varsity, was a guard. The Kees were very athletic looking, but not particularly big.

After high school I hadn't been to many college games. Now when I started going to Fort Valley games, I observed that most of the players here had average builds also — medium height if they were guards, and tall and skinny if they were forwards. But Walter Gilmore was different. Gilmore would grab the ball and thrust his big muscular arms and shoulders from side to side, intimidating the other team's players so they fell back. The 1969 season at FVSC was the first time I saw basketball played as the physical game it is today. Walter Gilmore was drafted in 1970 in the second round by the Portland Trailblazers and played for them for one season as a forward. Making game nights even better, our pep band played in the stands, and in addition to the cheerleaders, we had dancers perform at half-time on the court.

One night, I entered the gym through the doors on our side, as usual, for a game against our rival, Albany State College, another black college in the SIAC. The Albany fans arrived by bus, and they were streaming in through the set of doors to the visitors' side just as I came through to the home side.

"Honkey! Whitey! Fort Valley got a Honkey!" yelled some of the Albany fans when they saw me.

Some Fort Valley fans who knew me, and some who didn't, booed their rivals because of what they were yelling at me, "You wrong! No-o-o!"

At that moment, being supported like that, I felt like I belonged and like Fort Valley was my school.

19.

Anna and Ron Go to a Juke Joint

RON AND SCOTT both looked out for me during my first year at Fort Valley State College. Although we didn't think of ourselves this way, Scott and I were like two kids—young, just having received our master's degrees in English, and totally inexperienced in teaching. We also were new to life in a black community although Scott would have been more familiar with African Americans in his community since he was from Tennessee. Scott had moved to an apartment in Griffinline on Highway 96 after Dr. Brown put him out of the Dixon's house.

Ron was older but definitely new to the black community.

"I want to do for Mike and watch out for you," Ron explained while we sat in the kitchen of his new mobile home one afternoon. On the one hand, the Betty Friedan, *Feminine Mystique* side of me did not agree that I needed protecting. On the other hand, I looked forward to having hot dogs and beer at Lum's or going to Atlanta with Ron. The fact was, I hadn't even been able to get around until Ron helped me learn to drive, and, so far, I didn't have a female friend to do things with. I wasn't actually that independent.

Ron had shared what he considered to be a big mistake in his life that took place before he left Hawaii to attend graduate school at Kansas State. This may be what made him determined to be a protective friend but only a friend. Back then, he became close to the fiancé of his best friend, and the result was very bad. "I'm not going to have girlfriend or get married," he told me. "I don't want to be guilty anymore in life. I never forgive myself for breaking up my friend's marriage engagement in Hilo. That one reason why I went to Kansas."

Another firm position Ron took was that he would not accept any repayment or favors.

While I waited for him one evening to get ready to go out to dinner and to a club we'd heard about, I managed to calm the more ferocious one of his half-Siamese cats who had taken a swipe at me when I came in. When Ron came back in the kitchen, I said, "It's my turn to buy supper tonight, remember?"

"No, I pay, and I don't take nothing from people," Ron said. "I like to give. I don't want obligation."

He simply would not accept anything.

That night we planned to try a club we had heard about because I was still on a mission to hear live jazz. As early as grade school, and after hearing George Gershwin and Louis Armstrong, I developed a love of jazz. One thing that had excited me about accepting a job at a black college in the South, in the midst of black culture, was a hope to hear jazz live. It turned out to be less available than I thought. Thanks to George Holland's grants, I did eventually get to hear guest musicians on campus like the Cannonball Adderley Quartet and Donald Byrd. Duke Ellington appeared for a program in the gym, and much later I heard live music at Paschal's in Atlanta. This night, I convinced Ron that we should go to a black club, a "juke joint," to hear the music.

"I think we turn this way," Ron said.

It was evening and getting dark. We were on a two-lane road and saw dirt roads branching off it.

"Is this Crawford County or Taylor County?" I asked.

"Crawford, I think," said Ron. "Remember in Crawford we can buy beer and liquor. I'm not sure about Taylor."

We saw a lot of cars parked outside of a single-story frame building, and we could hear some drums and guitars coming from inside.

We parked and walked inside. It was a good thing we'd had supper first, because they weren't selling much except some pork skins and chips. And some "Co-Colas."

A man took our entrance money at the door.

"We BYOB here," he said.

On the outside, the club looked like it needed paint. The inside was a little nicer and contained a counter, some tables and chairs, and a small dance floor. The band was set up on one side. They weren't playing jazz, but soul music and the blues. I liked it; I thought the music was great.

As a couple—a relatively tall young white woman and a short Asian male—we must have stood out, but it didn't seem like the other patrons paid much attention to us. We watched the other people dance, and I tapped my foot to the music, but neither one of us was inclined to get up and dance.

"We stay for a while since we drive out here," Ron said, and I agreed.

That was my first and last time in a nightclub out in the country in Georgia. Or anywhere, for that matter.

20.

Anna and Scott Attend Church

S COTT DIDN'T GO OUT to that club in the country with us, but he did accompany me to church. Being half-Swedish, I attended a Lutheran church regularly when I lived with my family. After I moved to Madison to go to the university, I pretty much only went when I was worried about final exams. Scott and I decided to try the church across the street from the college, St. Luke's Episcopal.

"I'm going to go to St. Luke's with Scott Lewis," I mentioned to Miss Douglas in her office one day during the week before we planned to worship there.

I didn't go so far as to tell Miss Douglas that, based on a little bit of skepticism and some of my reading, I thought I was more of a Deist than an evangelical Christian. But I was still conservative enough to see value in the church tradition. Christianity insists on loving one another and on the equal value of every soul. Like the hymn says, "His eye is on the sparrow,...so I know he watches me."

In parts of the world touched by Christianity, I thought, rights are considered to be God-given, not given by a monarch or ruler, and all individuals are considered to be loved by God. At that time, I knew about the Crusades and other not-so-peaceful actions by Christian nations or groups, but I knew less about iniquities of Christian churches in America.

"I attend St. Luke's," said Miss Douglas. "Did you know that when we were the Fort Valley High and Industrial School, we were supported by the Episcopal Church?"

"You mean we weren't always a state school?"

"We learn on Founders Day that we were founded by a group of men, both white and black. Some were from up North. But then Episcopalians from Ohio and some from New York began to support the school. For a while, before we became a state college, we were part of a diocese in Georgia."

All this was news to me.

"There is also a white Episcopal church in Fort Valley, St. Andrew's," Miss Doulas added.

It bothered me to learn that black and white Episcopalians worshipped separately. I remembered that Dr. Henry Berry, one of the more vocal faculty members at our meetings, reported several times on his attempts to participate in services at the white Methodist church and other white churches in town. He said men stood at the door and asked him not to come in. As a member of the NAACP, he also reported on other civil rights activities when blacks were not treated fairly or did not receive due process. He referred to this so often that our colleagues gave him the nickname "Dr. Due Process."

I had no interest in going to St. Andrews. St. Luke's Episcopal Church is right across the street from the front gate of the college and the neon sign. In addition to Miss Douglas who attended St. Luke's, although she was not an Episcopalian, other colleagues from the college went there, including the coach, the registrar, some in the business offices, and several education professors along with school-teachers in the surrounding area. Later, I learned that the church was originally named the College Center, and it was established as an Episcopal mission after Fort Valley High and Industrial School became Fort Valley State College.

The American Church Institution agreed to let Fort Valley High and Industrial School be transferred to the state on the condition that a church would be available to the school. This was the point at which St. Luke's Episcopal Church was born. The College Center became St. Luke's.

Not counting Scott and me, all those who attended were black. Father Ramcharam was the vicar before I came, and he lived in the vicarage attached by a covered walkway to the parish hall of the church. But in 1968, there was no vicar in charge, which meant that morning prayer, rather than a communion service, was celebrated every Sunday. A male vestry member led the service.

St. Luke's is a simple red brick gothic structure with no separate entrance area or vestibule. Inside the door are wood pews on both sides of an aisle leading up to the altar. At the end of the aisle. one step up leads to the choir section, the lectern for scripture readings, and the pulpit where sermons are preached. The altar table stands at the back with room for the celebrant behind it.

A beautiful stained-glass window featuring a strong-looking Jesus surrounded by little children looks over the baptismal font. All the other windows were a clear textured glass, and there was no tapestry hanging behind the altar as there is now. Miss Douglas may have been the first woman ever to be asked to read scripture lessons during the service. Ladies in the church, except me most of the time, wore hats, and Miss Douglas deferred to that custom by placing a lace handkerchief on top of her head.

Old pictures show long lines of students streaming across the street from the campus and through the front doors of the church. Most of them were raised in Baptist, Christian Methodist Episcopal (CME), African Methodist Episcopal (AME) or Pentecostal churches. Before I arrived, students were required to attend church. Now that the college was not supposed to serve *in loco parentis*, the students' motivation to cross the street and attend this nearby church was greatly reduced.

Down the street, Trinity Baptist Church was becoming socially active. For example, the church was active in the civic life of the city and involved in such civil rights activities as voter registration, and it successfully recruited college students. All in all, the Episcopal Church with its reputation of light-skinned members and worshippers did not resonate with the students. I once heard someone from Savannah say that there was a test to enter the black Episcopal church there—the person's skin color should not be darker than the pecan wood framing the church's doors. That may be a myth, but in 1968–69, only a few students continued to worship at St. Luke's.

"I went to an Episcopal church at home," Scott murmured while we were waiting for the service to start.

"I always went to Lutheran churches," I whispered back. "But the one in Oshkosh was a high German church with kneelers and statues, so it was a little bit like this church. Women did not have to wear hats, though."

I did wear a black straw hat when we worshipped on Palm Sunday. Scott took a picture of me wearing that hat and a light green silk dress I sewed to wear on dressy occasions.

Another time, Scott asked me, "What poets did you like best while you were in college and grad school?" We were getting ready to go get something to eat, and I was waiting for him at his apartment in Griffinline.

"I haven't read too much modern stuff yet," I confessed. "I really like some of Wordsworth's poems and Browning's dramatic monologues."

"Have you read anything by Lawrence Ferlinghetti or Rod McKuen?" Scott asked.

I had, but their work seemed rather light to me compared to the poets I liked. Rod McKuen's seemed especially light.

"Ferlinghetti has some good ones. I could try to write some like that," I offered.

Just then, we heard a knock at Scott's door. It was a student, small in stature and dressed in a plain blue collared shirt and jeans. She looked at one of us and then the other.

"This is Brenda," Scott said. "She was one of my students in CEAP."

I knew CEAP was for students who weren't quite well-prepared enough for college, so I thought it was odd that the two of them would be hanging out.

"Scott livin' in my neighborhood, and I'm tellin' him about it," Brenda said. "I'm goin' in the Army next month, but he be all right."

Scott looked at me and kind of shrugged.

"You all goin' out?" Brenda wanted to know.

"We're just friends," I said, wondering if she knew I was married, and my husband was away in the Army himself.

"All right," she said. "Well, hope you get somethin' good to eat," and she let herself out, giving me the side eye.

"My student," Scott said sheepishly. "She lives around here and seems to think she's watching out for me."

It struck me that he might need someone to watch out for him. I also thought that if they became a couple, they'd be an odd one, especially because he was a Christian southern gentleman, not all that macho, and she was tough looking, not very feminine compared to any of my female friends.

21.

Arson and Influence

ALTHOUGH I DIDN'T have close female friends in Fort Valley yet, I was getting to know two new white people in the art department, Kay Shukair and Jeff Way, who was married to Jenny.

I went to Jeff and Jenny Way's house the first time with Mike when he was home from Fort Benning and visited them several other times after he was gone. They rented a small white frame house out in the country. Both of them were artists. Jenny was Jewish, from New York City. Jeff was from Ohio, and he sounded like my relatives on my mother's side from small towns in the Toledo area. Jeff taught in the art department at Fort Valley State College, and Jenny was volunteering to teach art at Hunt School and in an after-school program. Jenny was a bit taller than Jeff, who was average in height, and she had very curly, fine dark hair.

Paintings they had done hung all around their house, mostly abstracts in bright primary colors. Jeff's were geometric, and Jenny's were curvy. I wished I could have been an artist, and I admired their lifestyle and their talent. I still have the sketch Jenney used for one of her paintings. They also had a cat, always a plus for me.

Jenny talked about an art instructor she'd studied under.

"We worked on our pieces all semester," she said. "And then Mr. Court wanted to teach us a lesson about the importance of striving to improve as artists instead of congratulating ourselves over creations we'd already completed. He didn't want us to rest on our laurels. So, he had us all destroy the pieces we'd been working on. That was hard to do! But it was a good lesson, and I won't forget it."

It was strange and ironic, then, when a fire broke out and destroyed their rental house, their belongings, their artwork, everything but one cast iron skillet. We didn't say it, and it wasn't proven, but I believe now that it was arson. A Jewish New Yorker and a white man from the North teaching in a black college and living out in the country among white farms became a target for someone who didn't want integration and wanted to teach a lesson. I've had other experiences since then that solidify my belief that it was arson.

Gordon "Jack" Joyner, a successful son of black landowners in Fort Valley, offered to rent his vacant family home to the Ways who now had no place to live. One of Jeff's colleagues, Kay Shukair, who joined the art faculty during the year, signed on to help get the house ready. She was white, of Finnish ancestry, from Northern Wisconsin, and married to Ali, who was from Iran. Ali didn't come out there, but Kay and I and others helped the Ways assemble household items and clean up the Joyner house.

"I brought another broom," I said as I joined the others in the kitchen of the one-story house. "and I have some blue and white material so I can make curtains. I brought my tape measure."

"I don't know who was living here last," Kay said, wrinkling her nose. "Did you see the torn-up mattress on the floor in one of the bedrooms? There were mouse droppings. And what is that horrible brown stain?"

"You all might not see that up North," another helper said. "That's tobacco spit. They either chewed it or had snuff in their cheeks and spit it out."

But it was a fairly nice little house once we got it cleaned up and even painted a little. I hung the cheerful blue and white cotton curtains in the windows, and somebody donated a rug and other furniture. That house is just down the road from the Stallworth Trailer Park where I lived at the time and even closer to where I live today, half a century later, on the same road.

Jeff and Jenny appeared to survive the fire emotionally intact. She was prepared for the loss of her art by that art instructor a few years before. We grieved for their cat, which probably died in the fire since we never saw it again.

Near the end of the 1968–69 school year, Jeff and Jenny told me that they had decided not to stay.

"We believe that a black college ought to be able to develop or evolve based on its own culture and history," Jeff said. "We don't think white outsiders should try to influence its growth."

I thought it was interesting that they said that, especially because my father recently had won an award for a similar idea, that developing countries should use market research theory to determine their own needs, work force, and available materials rather than have American companies come in, build large factories, and take over their economies.

I stayed, though, and not just for one more year. I did take their advice to heart even though I couldn't resist offering ideas to my department, in faculty meetings, and even to student life administrators as time went on.

A shocking statement by another white faculty member also made an impression on me. Peter Dolce was a white English instructor who arrived in my first year at the college. Peter was from the Northeast somewhere. He was good-looking with curly black hair. I'd experienced arrogance like his at the University of Wisconsin from some New Yorkers. Peter tended to stay to himself.

But one day, when we happened to be the only two people in the office, he said to me, "I will talk to you when we are in here by ourselves, but not when other faculty or students are present, and not out on the campus. I don't want to be seen as someone who associates with white people."

I was taken aback. Peter was white. After Jeff's and Peter's comments, I still hung out with Ron and Scott and was friends with Jeff and Jenny and Kay, but I became conscious of my need to respect black culture instead of acting like I knew best.

In future years, I kept my place as an outsider who was there to help, as Instructor, then Assistant Professor, then Professor, instead of seeking promotions to administrative positions. (Thirty-six years later, in 2006, I did become Dean of Graduate Studies and Extended Education — the least important of the deans and a position that no longer exists.) I continued to make a point, over the years, of sitting with my black colleagues and friends instead of with groups of white faculty members. And the white faculty did tend to sit in groups. With my students, all of whom were black, on the other hand, I rarely thought about our respective racial identities.

22.

Grave-Digger Humor

I NTRODUCTION TO LITERATURE was my favorite class. I didn't
think much about racial identity when I was in my freshman and
sophomore classes. I was only four years older than the students, and
that made me feel a sense of camaraderie. But mainly, I was focused
on my mission: to help them learn to think.

Again, the textbooks selected by Miss Douglas made an enormous
difference in my ability to teach. *Literature in Critical Perspectives*,
edited by Walter K. Gordon, had the readings arranged so that different critical approaches could be learned and applied by the students.
Social (or sociological) criticism, formalist (or what we called "new")
criticism, psychological (or Freudian) criticism, archetypal (or Jung-
ian) criticism. The final unit in the book applied the four types, plus
a category of criticism called "Mixed," to one book, *Billy Budd, Sailor*
by Herman Melville. I learned about historical criticism in college
and graduate school, and sociological criticism was close to that. I
was already familiar with the others. I probably concentrated more
on interpreting the literature than on the critical perspectives, and
this was helped along by our supplementary text, a paperback titled
Writing about Literature by Bernard Cohen. It included explana-
tions and examples students could understand. The rubric I've used
to grade literature essays was derived from Cohen: students receive
30% for the thesis or interpretation, 30% for examples supporting
that interpretation, 20% for explanation of how the examples support
the interpretation, and 20% for usage and style. The rubric helped me
teach and helped me avoid being swayed by shows of intelligence.

I've always been a sucker for very intelligent students, even though discipline and hard work can lead to more success in the end. I was fortunate to begin teaching with the support of these texts.

Like most English classes, my Introduction to Literature class that spring was held in the Academic Building. We were upstairs, on the side of the building facing "The Yard" and across from Patton Hall, the music building. We kept the windows of the Academic Building open since there was no air conditioning. That meant we heard the lawn mowers outside, and, before the public schools were integrated, we heard band students practicing during a week in May. Fort Valley State College was known for Band Clinic, a gathering of bands from black high schools. Often, I would get drowned out by the sound right before I was about to make an important point in the lecture or discussion—or that's how it seemed. If it wasn't the bands, it was the lawnmowers.

We were in the sophomore literature class on one of those days, trying to discuss Shakespeare's *Hamlet* in between mower passes. The English majors in the Survey of British Literature classes still were a bit skeptical of me and hard to rouse, talking to each other more than they were listening or talking to me. But the sophomores in this literature class were the opposite. Some who thought they wouldn't like any English class started to get into it. Students in one class I'll always remember included Al Marcus Miller, the son of a campus janitor (who also was the descendant of a founder); his friend Melvin, a future physician; Diane Felton, a young woman from Montezuma I stayed in touch with; Joe Henry Lewis, who later died in a car accident and who was so clever he got As without coming to class all the time, and another sharp young man, John Paschal from Macon, who had a facial expression with a built-in grin. The students were lively, sharp, and engaged, and it was fun to be their instructor.

I had loved the lectures in my own college classes. Some of the lecturers, such as Karl Kroeber and Alvin Whitley in English, George L. Mosse in European history, and Ralph Andreano in economics, were phenomenal speakers and great minds whose ideas I still remember. Students who weren't even enrolled in their classes came just to hear the lectures. But I soon learned that lecture didn't work well for me. Discussion with bits of lecture interspersed worked better — in other words, the Socratic method.

One day, we discussed the grave-digging scene in *The Tragedy of Hamlet, King of Denmark* where Hamlet asks the grave digger whose grave it is that he is digging.

The man answers, "Mine, sir."

Hamlet responds with the words, "I think it be thine, indeed for thou liest in't." (5.1.122).

I chuckled at the pun. I looked out at the faces in my class and saw that only one other person, John Paschal, was chuckling, too. (Joe Henry Lewis was absent again.)

For some reason, the baffled looks on all the other faces struck me as funny, and I chuckled more. Midwestern humor, especially academic midwestern humor, and southern humor, especially black humor, simply are not the same. As I got to know students and others from Georgia, I learned that the morbid fact of being stuck with digging a grave would have been considered far more humorous than any quibble between two meanings of the word "lie."

After class that day, I talked to a few of the students and then went to the ladies' room on the first floor of the building located on the hall behind the stage. Thinking about the class I'd just finished, I stepped to the sink and looked at myself in the mirror. I had to blink. My white face and straight blondish hair startled me. I forgot I was different. What did my students think of me, a white woman from the North with a husband in the war?

I thought about Mike undergoing Special Forces training while I was in Fort Valley working, but interacting with my students kept my mind occupied in a good way.

23.

The Summer of 1969

MIKE COULDN'T take leave in the summer of 1969 since he was completing his training at Fort Bragg. I don't know if he even wanted to since he was very focused on becoming a Green Beret. I was a very new driver, but I was driving, and I even had the nerve to drive to and in Atlanta. Interstate 75 wasn't completed yet, so I would have taken US highway 341 to get to Atlanta.

I went there one week to meet my little sister who had been accepted to a summer program in French at the University of Georgia. We went shopping, had a meal, and went to a movie. I was driving on Ponce de Leon Avenue in the area of the old Sears, when suddenly the traffic light turned yellow. So, of course, being a good citizen, I stopped. The driver of the city bus behind me was accustomed to driving through the yellow, as evidently all Atlanta drivers are, and he was taken completely by surprise. When he swung to the left to avoid hitting me in the rear end, he hit a car that was to the left of me.

I thought fast and turned up a sloping driveway on the right and into the Sears parking lot.

"What are you going to do?" Nancy wondered. She usually was calm to the extreme, but she looked a bit concerned.

"I don't know. I guess I'll just wait until the police finish examining the accident," I said.

So, we waited.

During her short visit, Nancy, who is six years younger than me, told me that she had decided to stay at home after high school graduation because she would be needed to take care of our parents. I was baffled when I heard that since I hadn't learned of any illnesses or problems from their letters. I wrote home to inquire about it, and my dad just said that Mom had been suffering with a cold. With Vietnam on the horizon in my own life, I didn't pursue the issue any farther.

After Nancy went back to Wisconsin, Mike said his training schedule allowed him more flexibility, and he came to Fort Valley and got the VW fastback to use in North Carolina. I wanted to keep driving, so I bought a used VW beetle, a dark green one, probably a 1965 model based on the style of bumper it had.

I signed a contract to teach the coming year at the rank of Assistant Professor. I forgot about the plan to stay in Georgia for only a year. But I wasn't teaching summer school, so I drove up to see Mike at Fort Bragg for two consecutive weekends. The second time I was run off the road by an old man who didn't look both ways as he drove out of a shopping center into the highway. I remember that other drivers waved at me in sympathy. After that, we decided to rent one-half of a small trailer in Fayetteville, and I brought Pokey and Fu with me to go and stay with Mike before he would be deployed to Vietnam.

The few weeks there were surreal. I felt very emotional and needy. Mike focused on his training and went to sleep quickly every night. Then I got a urinary tract infection that sent me to the infirmary where they gave me pills that caused me intense itching from head to toe for over a day.

But it was good to be together. When it was time for me to go back to Fort Valley, or rather for both of us to go in order to get the two cars back, Mr. Fu escaped from the trailer. We walked around in the dark calling his name. Fu apparently sat there watching us look for him, but he finally emerged and the next morning we were able to get going. Mike may have left from Fort Benning or the Atlanta Airport near the end of the summer to start his tour in Vietnam. My memory of that time is a blur.

I celebrated my twenty-fourth birthday on August 13, 1969. At the end of the summer, probably the beginning of September before the college year started in those days, my mom, my dad, and my brother Peter came to visit, and we all went to Jekyll Island. We had grown up going to northern lakes (except for my mom's main fishing place, the Maumee River in Ohio). The ocean was a whole new level of fun in the water even though Dad and Peter got stung by jelly fish.

My family came partly to give me support, I'm sure. Mike and I began to keep in touch through letters, and I worried.

YEAR TWO:
1969–1970

24.

Year Two Begins

I N MID-SEPTEMBER, I returned to work and to my desk in the English office. We didn't interview students for the Scope Chart anymore, but I advised a few English majors and had conferences with students from my classes who seemed to need help. At my request, Miss Douglas had assigned me five classes, instead of the usual four, which on the quarter system met three hours per week. After a whole year of teaching, I now felt confident and established in the job.

What was called the Vietnam Conflict since Congress had not declared war showed no signs of abating. An extraordinary number of shocking events had already occurred. In the spring of 1968, before I arrived in Georgia, the Rev. Martin Luther King, Jr., and Robert F. Kennedy were assassinated. There was violence at the Democratic National Convention. The National Organization for Women (NOW) protested for women's rights in New York and other places. The Supreme Court made the decision mandating public school desegregation at long last, and Students for a Democratic Society (SDS) held a sit-in at Harvard.

And man landed on the moon.

As Fall 1969 got started, anti-war demonstrations continued in various places and the lottery for the draft was instituted, to answer inequities in the draft system. Yet, despite the national climate, the school year at Fort Valley State College started out fairly calmly for me. To make my life more complete, I finally made a good female friend.

As the number of students coming to college increased, the college hired more faculty. Scott had left after one year, and Betty Stokes was hired in his place to work in CEAP and part-time in the English Department. Betty made good friends in CEAP, including Lorette and Dortha and Maggie, and she and I also struck up a friendship. She was my first, and became my best, female friend who was near to my age.

Betty's older boyfriend lived out of state. She called him "my friend." He came to see her frequently, but she usually was available to go shopping with me and just talk. Betty had a serene beauty—large eyes, a warm smile, long hair. And she was always very direct in her observations about people (including me). When we went to a store (there were no malls), I constantly had to stop and wait for her because I couldn't get used to walking as slowly as she did, and she couldn't get used to walking as fast as I did. Betty had type I diabetes, so everywhere we went, she chose mixed nuts as her snack, and she drank diet sodas. She kept wrapped pieces of candy on hand in case her sugar dropped.

We didn't do anything big and exciting. Mostly we looked for clothes at women's stores and talked about our colleagues. Mainly, we just talked. And as my family observed, I like to talk.

Despite her more languid approach to life, Betty did agree to go with me to football games sometimes, and there we sat and observed people as much as we watched the game.

"My friend is coming to the game this weekend," she said one afternoon at my place. "You can sit with us."

Switching subjects and looking at one of her bracelets, she said, "You know that sociology professor, Dr. Morton, is trying to talk to me." (That isn't his real name.) She gave an amused smile.

"Is his office in Peabody?" I asked. "I haven't met him yet. He looks sharp!"

"Jan and I are going over to Arrah Moore's house tonight," Betty said, changing subjects again. "Jan lives at her mother's house, and she can't drink there."

"Oh," I said. "Arrah and her husband go to St. Luke's. But Episcopalians don't have any rules against drinking."

Betty asked if I had received a letter from Mike lately. "I got one last week," I said. "It's hard for me to see what it's like over there in Vietnam. I don't think he can say much about it, especially since the Special Forces are doing things that are not in the news." But I didn't talk that much about Mike. I just knew he was supposed to be back in about a year.

Betty drank her Diet-Rite and I finished my Seven-Up. Then we headed to Macon to eat supper and shop. Before we went into the department store in Macon, Betty always stopped to buy a small package of mixed nuts at the shop next door. Then we'd go to Davison's women's section and try on outfits. One time she chose a dark paisley top and a straight knee-length skirt while I flirted with a mini-skirt but decided against it.

"I have this Vogue pattern for a dress," I said on the way back to Fort Valley, "and did you see my silk catalog? I love silk. I remember one silk dress my mother had; she let me wear it when I got older. It was black and taupe paisley. I'm going to order some more of that silk fabric from Thailand."

I don't know how she came to be that way, but Betty never seemed to discriminate by race, although she was willing to share gossip with anyone. Lorette and I were white, and Dortha and Maggie were black. Lorette loved acting. Surprisingly, since Betty was not an extrovert, she had done some acting in college too, which I had not. Betty didn't ever characterize a person of her own race as "acting white," and she didn't make remarks I've heard from other black people such as, "That's what happens when you work with black."

Other new people joined us in our English faculty office. Maybe that's the reason Miss Douglas moved me later, to make room. But while I was still there, hanging out with JC, Mrs. Cook, and Mrs. Adams, I made friends with a new white English instructor who came from Tennessee via Iowa State's creative writing program. His name was Mike Murphy. His friends and I called him Murphy. He wasn't any older than me, and his wife Suzanne was younger. Murphy, Mrs. Cook, and I joked quite a bit, especially when we were the only ones in the office. Although Mrs. Cook probably was ten years older than me, she had a practical streak and viewed the foibles of others with a good sense of humor. My desk was still in the middle, with Murphy on my left and Sadie Malone to my right, and the three of us facing Mrs. Cook.

One afternoon, Murphy and I talked about how we tricked our students into doing their reading before class. Mrs. Cook listened to our conversation.

"I make them answer questions about random pages so they have to read all of *Oedipus* in order to know what's going on at that exact point," I said. "I've got a few who are really on top of things. Some of them don't always come to class, though."

"I just make them do writing on a surprise question," Murphy said.

"It's a constant battle," Mrs. Cook said. "Don't give up!"

Murphy and Mrs. Cook packed up to go home at that point. I finished recording the last of my grades, and I went home to an empty Buddy the Mobile Home.

25.

Speaking Up

D ISCUSSIONS IN our faculty meetings rarely made reference
to events outside our college life. During the meetings
we debated and voted on new courses or programs or tweaks in
registration processes. I didn't know where the policies we voted into
existence were printed except those that ended up in the *Bulletin*.

It wasn't until later, when I went to Kent State in 1972 to do a PhD
program, that it really occurred to me: nothing regarding governance
seemed to be written at FVSC. At the graduate school at Kent State,
the English Department and the graduate college had rules and a
written constitution. I was elected one year to be a graduate student
representative, which gave me half a vote at faculty meetings.

At Fort Valley State, in contrast, it appeared to me all proto-
cols and policies were based on tradition. To know how to handle
something, it was necessary to ask someone how it was done. The
college catalog, the *Bulletin*, listed requirements for graduation, and
I knew about the Scope Chart. But hiring requirements, faculty
governance, rights and responsibilities, vacation and time off, sick
leave — if these were written down, I was not aware of it. Today, Fort
Valley State University has the *Faculty Handbook*, a constitution, a
mission statement, and University System of Georgia (USG) and
Southern Association of Colleges and Schools (SACS) requirements
as well as requirements and standards for other accrediting associa-
tions. We have federal student aid and GI Bill requirements, National
Association of Athletics requirements, and so forth. In my first four
years at FVSC, we debated matters at faculty meetings and seemed

to decide them there. President Blanchet presided, and Dean Banks assisted. During summers, the meetings continued with Registrar, Houser Miller, presiding along with C.W. Pettigrew, the director of the graduate school.

Today, doing business without policies, job descriptions, and evaluation procedures would lead to lawsuits and votes of no confidence against the administration. In the late sixties, I felt that we respected our own aristocracy's leadership. It was all we knew, and that was comforting, to me in my twenties, as an instructor first and then as an assistant professor.

This did not mean the faculty meetings were quiet.

We usually met in a wide room on the second floor of the Hunt Library, which is now the Bywaters Building. The windows had the same malfunctioning venetian blinds found in the other buildings, and the faculty sat in chairs used by the students when we weren't meeting. The president, the secretary, and the dean were at tables in the front.

At one of these meetings, Dr. Blanchet called upon Dr. Henry Berry again. Dr. Berry was tall and portly and always wore a nice suit. His voice was always a bit high-pitched and hoarse.

"I visited the First Methodist Church on last Sunday," he informed us loudly. "We must keep trying to integrate the house of the Lord in this community. We must also demand our rights at all businesses. Were you denied service at any church or business in Fort Valley? All of us must demand due process when our rights are trampled."

He sat down, and other faculty members murmured approval though no one else spoke up. We admired Dr. Berry (Dr. Due Process) for his activism and his work with the NAACP. That didn't keep his colleagues from giving him a new nickname after the visit to our campus of Adam Clayton Powell.

Powell spoke to a huge audience in the Woodward Gymnasium. I watched from a seat high up in the stands, fascinated to see someone from television in real life. I don't recall the text of Powell's speech, though it must have been on voting rights. Dr. Berry sat only a little lower in the stands than my position, and he stood up after Powell's speech to ask a question.

He began by stammering, "D-d-does you—"

People laughed, and after that he was dubbed, "Dr. Does You" instead of "Dr. Due Process."

In the faculty meeting, which was later, we continued to hear about voting rights. A student life employee, the Rev. Julius Simmons, stood up and shared news about the coming election. Dr. Banks was running for County Commissioner, and if he was elected, he would be the first black person to hold office in Peach County. Rev. Simmons's church, Trinity Baptist, was the site of organized activity to insure voting rights for black people in Fort Valley and Peach County.

But not all faculty concerns were so noble. Dr. Gupta stood up in this meeting (as he did in every meeting) to complain just for the sake of complaining—or maybe so he would get recognition, too. Dr. Gupta was short and slight of build with shoulders bigger than the rest of him. His chiseled features and dark-framed glasses as well as his Hindi accent and the volume of his delivery made all his statements emphatic.

"Advisement should not be on days that faculty are not scheduled to teach!" Dr. Gupta said.

Dr. Bellamy, who had just returned from having earned his PhD in history, gave a succinct response. "Faculty are on the clock September 1st," he said, ending the discussion.

Wilma Anderson had an announcement about the library, although the head librarian was Miss Homie Regulus, not Miss Anderson.

"Please remind students to return books they check out so that others can use them. And faculty must put books and articles on reserve if they are assigned to classes," she reminded us.

As I observed her plain dress and hair and listened to her blunt way of speaking, I remembered that she had once been in the Women's Army Corps. I could picture her in that uniform.

"Thank you, Miss Anderson," replied Dr. Blanchet.

I am not known for keeping my mouth shut. And now I had a year's experience as a college instructor under my belt. I raised my hand. When I was recognized, I said, "Can we please develop a better registration process so that students do not have to carry cards from one place to another and they can get in the classes they need to graduate? Sometimes the ones who don't need the classes get there first, and then the seniors and juniors have to get special permission to be added to classes or else delay their graduation."

I knew this because I helped sign students' cards during registration. I also remembered that I had similar problems at UW. I had to ask permission to get into Alvin Whitley's Late Victorian Prose class when I was a master's student because I had never been able to carry my card up the hill to Bascom Hall in time to get in when I was an undergraduate.

"We will look into the problem, Professor Mitchell," answered Dr. Blanchet.

I walked to the mailbox that afternoon, my mind occupied by students, classes, and my role as a faculty member. A letter from my dad was in the box, but nothing from Mike this time. He couldn't really say that much in his letters, but I still hoped I'd get another one soon.

26.

Talking with Scientists

T HE DAY AFTER the faculty meeting, I went over to Ron's office. We planned to go to Lum's in Macon again for supper. Ron worked in the Tabor Agriculture Building. His office was very small, but at least he had an office to himself, probably because he was a researcher and had his PhD. All offices of the Division of Agriculture and their auditorium were in Tabor, and Tabor was connected to Miller by a hall and a short stairway. Coming up those steps and going into Miller, the first offices you would see belonged to the Head of the Division of Math and Science, Dr. William Moorehead. The faculty members I met in the Miller/Tabor Building were all men: Dr. Moorehead, Mr. George Canty, Mr. Harvey Bannister, Dr. Robert Steele, Dr. Earnest Corker, Dr. David Eaton, Dr. Stanley Kroman, Dr. Cyril Brown, Mr. Leroy Combs. They were humorous characters, constantly joking. All were black except Dr. Kroman, who was a chemistry professor, and one agriculture professor, Dr. Stanley Jacklyn, both of whom were white. In addition, there were people from India in Agriculture, including Dr. Syed Raman. Dr. Raman was a friend of Ron's. Actually Dr. Raman, Dr. Kroman, and Dr. Jacklyn weren't that humorous.

Ron's was the last office, next to the back door of the Tabor Building. To go from his office to the front of the building, you turned down a hall that had one or two more offices or supply rooms and a big cooler or meat locker. Ron and I headed down this white-painted hall towards the place where Tabor connected with Miller. We passed Dr. Stallworth, who happened to be standing in the hall.

"How's it going?" Dr. Stallworth asked, seeming to be directing the question to me. By now, both Ron and I were his trailer park tenants.

"Great, thank you," I responded. I had a question about the meat locker we'd just passed, but Dr. Stallworth looked like he was busy, so I held my thought.

We made a right turn, went up the two or three steps, and entered the row of offices belonging to the Biology Department. Ron needed to submit some paperwork for a general biology class he had been tagged to teach along with his animal science classes. Dr. Moorehead was in his office, and he said what he always said to me and others:

"Well, hello there, Mis Um-um-um..."

"Mitchell," I said, although I knew perfectly well that he remembered my name. "Dr. Moorehead," I said, "I was wondering what happens to the meat that Agriculture stores in that cooler in the Tabor Building."

"Used to take it to the dining hall to feed the students," he answered. "Some federal rule against doing that now. You looking to get some steaks?"

I knew by his grin that he was joking, as usual, at least about the steaks.

As we left, Ron said, "That a waste, why don't the college give it to some people?"

Next, we ran into George Canty, whose office was in the Chemistry Department upstairs. He was downstairs delivering something to the division office. Canty was working on his doctorate through Nova University, which was located in Florida. He was a joker, too.

"What you doing this week with all that federal money, Abe [pronounced A-be]?" Canty asked.

I already knew that the University of Georgia, an 1895 land grant institution, was holding back funds the government had designated for Fort Valley State College's agricultural program that we should have had since we were also an 1895 land grant.

"Doc's building barn for all that cattle," Ron joked in return. Dr. Stallworth, Dr. Raman, and Ron all were trying to do research on a shoestring at this time.

"You need to give me some of that money!" Canty said.

Besides the fact that Canty was going to Nova, and Clinton Dixon was going to graduate school in Oklahoma, Dr. Steele, a physical science professor, had just returned from Wyoming. The State of Georgia offered funding for black faculty in the University System of Georgia to earn their degrees out of state so it would not have to admit them to a university in Georgia. Most science professors as well as some in other areas got PhDs from out of state, most commonly from Ohio State. A few humanities professors chose to go to Atlanta University, a black private institution in Atlanta.

I'm not sure where Dr. Jacklyn and his wife were from, but they were not local. Dr. Jacklyn was a researcher in plant science. I made one of my first and only forays into political/philosophical conversation when I went with Ron to a party at the Jacklyns' house. (This was not a party like at Rufus and Mary's, with drinking and dancing, but mainly one where people sat around, ate, and talked.)

I tried to explain to Dr. Jacklyn and his wife why I was against the military draft. We sat on their patio enjoying grilled hot dogs and hamburgers. Dr. Jacklyn said something about how the fighting seemed to be getting worse in Vietnam and the US was sending more ammunition, planes, guns, and recruits.

With that opening, I tried sharing my viewpoint. "We are supposed to be fighting communism, but our government also is using coercion when young men are forced against their will to go into the military and even fight in the war."

"I don't know about that," Jacklyn said, with a look of discomfort on his face.

"Not only are they pursuing a war that is killing American soldiers," I said, not taking my first clue, "but they even imprison men who refuse to go. I have a friend from Texas who was in prison for that."

Dr. Jacklyn looked even more uncomfortable, and Mrs. Jacklyn got up to offer food to some of the other guests.

Uh-oh, I said to myself. I might have been going for the shock value to some extent, but I realized that they were alarmed and confused by my ideas. I had already had similar discussions with Ron, who was a conservative like my dad and who, as a Japanese-American, felt strongly about his patriotism. But Ron did not get upset or uncomfortable; he just told me when he did not agree.

Except for Ron, I rarely interacted with researchers like Dr. Jacklyn, and I wasn't in the habit of discussing political subjects with colleagues. In my literature studies, I had come across the philosophy of Associationism. I understood it to mean that no two people view the world the same because we associate what we perceive based on different experiences. Looking through that lens, I knew I should be careful what I shared and how I interpreted others.

27.

Mishaps

W HETHER AT social gatherings or on campus, I thought of myself as an idealistic, serious professional. But I often ended up being awkward, whether it was on campus or off.

Now I was in my second year of teaching and having my own desk in the faculty office. After seeing an ad for a John Lennon book bag (an English school-boy bag or messenger bag), I ordered one to carry my papers and books. It was gray with a flap and shoulder strap. I felt at home now at Fort Valley State College, but I was still aware of being looked at because I was young, female, and white.

One day, I parked my car in one of the angled spaces across from the Academic Building, hung my book bag and my homemade Indian cotton purse over my shoulder, and looked for a break in the traffic in order to cross the road. Students on the other side of the road walked to and from the Academic Building and along the sidewalk between the large azalea bushes. The traffic consisted of cars heading to spots in front of the building or to parking spots across from the student center or farther down near the stadium parking lot.

I saw a break in the traffic, stepped out quickly — and then I tripped and fell. I felt my face turn red, clashing with my blue striped, brown turtleneck and brown knit mini-skirt. I got up and grabbed my bags as fast as I could.

"I'm OK! I'm fine!" I said to the students who offered to assist me, and I hurried into the building.

Not long after that, Ron suggested that we go to Atlanta to a steak house he'd heard about. It wasn't a Japanese steak house, but he wanted to try it. When we arrived at the large, dimly lit restaurant, we learned that we were too early. They were not going to seat guests at the tables or take dinner orders until after five thirty. However, the bar was open, so we decided to have a drink while we waited.

"You ever have a Manhattan?" Ron asked.

"I haven't had very many mixed drinks," I answered as I leaned my elbows on the leather-topped bar. "My dad likes martinis, and I found out I like those, with an olive. When I was at Oshkosh, and I wasn't really at drinking age yet, I tried some rum and ginger ale. This man who was acting like our mentor drank old-fashioneds. They're made with whiskey. I don't know if I ever tried one."

"I'm getting Manhattan," Ron said. "I get one for you, too."

When we'd finished our drinks (on empty stomachs), the tables still weren't ready, so we both had another. Then I excused myself to go to the ladies' room. As I opened the door to the stall inside, I experienced the sensation that there were two of me, one watching and commenting on the other.

Now she is opening the door. Now she is closing the door. Now she is turning the water on. Now she is washing her hands.

I remembered what Mike always said. I wasn't very experienced. I don't think I've had another Manhattan since.

My lack of experience in driving was still showing, too. Paul Rehling, the mayor of Fort Valley at the time, was making changes in the city. South Macon Street, the street leading to the college and beyond to middle class black neighborhoods and then our trailer park, was widened to create three lanes all the way to the entrance to the college, one of which was a middle lane. People lost a large part of their front yards to this project. The middle was for turning only, but I got behind a slow truck on the way to the college from town one day and decided to pass by using the middle lane. Bingo. I got pulled over by the city police and got a ticket.

I thought this was unreasonable, so I looked for a way to get the ticket resolved. It turned out that Mr. Rehling also was the city judge, so I went to see him. He was very gracious and tore the ticket up.

Naturally, that made him seem to me like a very good person. Mayor Rehling owned a radio station, served five terms as mayor, and was known in later years for his leadership in restoring the main street in Fort Valley after a tornado came through.

That ticket incident was only one problem I had as an inexperienced driver on South Macon Street. A new curb had been installed on the turn to Carver Drive with a storm sewer opening below it. When I made a turn onto Carver Drive, I got too close to the high curb and got my little Volkswagen stuck on it. Friendly passers-by on the college side of town helped lift my car off the curb so I could be on my way, another example of how those in the black neighborhood made me feel welcome.

28.

Kick-Off

I CAME TO Fort Valley State with the mindset that college is for the cultivation of ideas and obtaining knowledge and that sports are a distraction, or certainly not essential. It didn't take long for me to revert to my Wheaton Community High School Pep Club days and understand that a school needs spirit and good morale. Football and basketball games fostered a sense of community just as they did for me and my friends back when I was in high school, especially at Wheaton.

The students, and most faculty, were excited as the 1969 football season began. The Wildcats football team was excellent as usual. In the fifties, we pep club members and all the students in my high schools followed the rules of supporting our team, participating in cheers, being a good sport, and standing up for every kick-off. In contrast, the fans in the stands at FVSU yelled and complained at their own team, criticized the coaches, and booed the referees. Others hooted, slapped each other's hands, and, pretending to fall over, found everything hilarious. These were usually the ones who had brought paper bags containing their own drinks, in flasks or simply in bottles.

Football games also were a fashion show. In this era of Superfly, the men were as much a fashion show as the women. Some of the men wore sleeveless jumpsuits over shirts with puffed sleeves and "skys," or large-brimmed hats on their heads. Some had to choose between wearing their carefully combed-out and sculptured afros or wearing their hats. The less extravagant men dressed in gray or light brown double-knit wool sweaters worn outside the pants, falling just below the belt.

A protest actually occurred the next year, after integration, when the school board—which was all white, of course, and appointed, not elected—tried to enforce a dress code with a rule against sweaters or shirts being worn without being tucked in. The rule clearly seemed to be aimed at a style worn only by well-dressed black males. To me, it really was a shame. I knew that being nicely dressed was important to the students. They even took their jeans to the laundry to be starched and pressed with a crease down the front and back of each leg.

At the games, both the Superflys and the double-knit sweater-wearers liked boots, usually with slightly raised heels. The women dressed up in wide-leg pants or skirts and boots. Now that I was in Georgia, not the casual Midwest, I tried to step it up a bit and wear matching pants and tops instead of school t-shirts and jeans. A blue corduroy outfit the Fort Valley cleaners ruined by washing and starching it instead of dry-cleaning it was one of my attempts.

On game day we stood in line to buy a ticket at the gate, walked around to the end of the field to the home side, and tried to find a seat that was not too high up but with a view of the field that was not blocked by the fans parading back and forth. After we took our seats (and while late-comers continued to come in), an ROTC color guard brought in the United States flag, and we stood to sing the "Star-Spangled Banner." I always stood up for the kick-off at the beginning of the game, but I gave it up on subsequent kick-offs since no one else was doing it. The fans more-or-less responded to the cheerleaders although the buzz of conversation among the fans was just about as loud as the sound of cheering. Despite the joking and criticizing, the fans were very loyal. We always clapped and sang together the song, "I'm so glad I go to Fort Vall-ee!"

The half-time program was impressive. All the opposing schools still went to the trouble and expense of bringing their own bands. The other school's band would play first, usually facing us, but sometimes facing the visitors' side, and our band would play next. Each band's program began with marching and playing in formation, including one formation spelling out the initials of the school. At one point in every performance, everyone on the field threw down the instruments and danced, including some of the heavier band members who would manage to get a laugh.

Someone should write a book on the history of football at Fort Valley State College. I tried as hard as I could to see the plays made in the games by my students, including Toledo (Cedric King), Lovett Frank Redding, Samuel Covington, Paul Andrews, Ronnie Mells, and many others.

I've taught so many football players that it is hard to remember who was playing in what year and whether they played under Coach Lomax or Coach Porter who came later. The legendary coach, L.J. "Stan" Lomax was greatly respected by all, and he behaved in a humble, up-right manner. He and his family, Mary Lucille and their three children, went to St. Luke's. Coach, as we called him, was tall and light-skinned, originally from Brunswick, near where the Henrys were from, but the Lomaxes were not Geechee. He coached some of the other sports in addition to football.

I do recall that, especially before and after half-time, it got hard to see the plays in the game because those with new clothes strolled back and forth in front of us, conversing with each other and with their acquaintances in the stands. I didn't really mind. It helped me keep up with all the latest fashions.

29.

Some White Folks

BETTY AND I had spent some time with a new female faculty
member in English, Camille Willingham. One thing we did
was to go and eat together at a café opened by an art instructor,
Delearn Allen. The café was across the tracks, but just across, so its
clientele consisted of black townspeople, faculty, and a few students.

In the English faculty office after a late afternoon class one day,
Camille and I started talking about what to wear to work. Camille
was as tall as me. On that particular day, she was wearing a skirt
and a blouse.

"I don't want to get too dressed up," I said. (I happened to be wearing a skirt and blouse that day also.) "It seems like we're supposed
to wear skirts or dresses. But sometimes I want to wear pants, even
bell-bottom pants."

"I know what you mean," Camille said. "I need to buy some things
since I just started teaching. Is there any place around here?"

"There's Par-San," I said. "And Khoury's is better. Their clothes
are a little more up to date or for younger women. After I had my
ears pierced, I started making earrings out of copper wire and beads.
Lorraine Khoury has my earrings for sale in her store."

By this time, we were packing up to leave the Academic Building.
I slung my John Lennon book bag over my shoulder, and we started
out past the azalea bushes that were on both sides of the sidewalk
leading from the front door of the building. As we headed to our
cars, I said, "Let's go look at Khoury's Women's store. I want to get
something with pants I can wear to games and to work. Want to
ride with me downtown?"

"Well, OK," said Camille. "They might have something for me."
We got in my car together and headed down South Macon Street and across the tracks to town. Thinking we might look in Par-San's, too, I parked at the beginning of the block on Main Street in front of a bank and across from Par-San's and Avera Drug.

The stores downtown looked like those in most American small towns—two story, brick, with flat fronts and roofs and maybe some ornamental cement work at the first-floor level and along the roof lines. We got out of my car and started walking towards Khoury's when we noticed the doors of several stores open and some white customers and workers step outside to stare at us. I didn't know if Camille sensed this, too, but I was sure they were staring because we were a young white woman and a young black woman, strangers in town, walking together as equals.

When we got to Khoury's, I quietly asked Camille, "Did you see those people looking at us?"

"Yeah," Camille said. She smiled sadly and said, "It be's that way sometime."

I've heard that expression again and again, humorous and fatalistic. That was the day I got a double-knit pants outfit. And I got another lesson about the South.

I also experienced, saw, and heard about troubling things related to medical services. When I developed bronchitis after suffering from a cold or allergies, I went to a doctor in town, Dr. Nathan. The Nathans probably were the only Jewish family in town. (The Khourys were Lebanese.) He was a good doctor, and over the years, he and his wife donated generously to the community.

I found Dr. Nathan's office, which was off Vineville Street, about a half mile from Dr. Palms's house. It was right around the corner from the Vineville neighborhood, but it wasn't actually in the area where black people lived.

I entered the waiting room and saw two rows of seats on my left with a sign saying "White" and two rows on my right with a sign saying "Colored." A few people, separated by race, were sitting on each side. When I got over my shock, I did what I hope any white twenty-four-year-old from the North would have done. I went in and sat down on a chair on the Colored side.

Later, visiting with Maybelle again, I brought this up.

"I guess all the doctors' offices in Georgia are segregated," I said.

"That not a big deal," Maybelle answered matter-of-factly. "But they was a baby born in the Fort Valley hospital with you know, no hole in its bottom."

"No anus?" I said.

"The baby almost die before they find out."

"But that's where they take a baby's temperature," I protested. "They should have found that out in the first hour!"

"And a accident with black in Byron," Maybelle continued. Byron was the other city in Peach County. "They didn't send no ambulance 'til it was too late."

I knew this was hearsay, but I readily believed it. From then on, and for decades, both in protest against the inequitable treatment of black people and because I didn't trust local medical standards, I went to Macon for all of my doctor's appointments.

30.

"Mrs. Mitchell looks like a Texian."

ONE QUARTER, I required all the students in my freshman English classes to write thirty-five-page autobiographies. I gave this assignment because I believed that doing some extensive writing would make the students better writers. In the end, I probably was more affected by their autobiographies than the students were as I developed insights into their lives.

One young woman I'll call Lorna Register had curvature of the spine and carried a large pocketbook to sit on and enable her to use classroom chairs. She wrote of traveling with her parents who were migrant workers through several southern states while she was growing up. Many years later, I had a young black woman with a doctorate as a colleague who had the same problem as Lorna, curvature of the spine. I was graduate dean, and this young professor reported to one of the department heads in the graduate school. She objected to her supervisor's instructions, especially about how to teach online, and left in the middle of a semester. I thought back to Lorna and wondered if this young professor had also had difficult experiences and how they had affected her.

One day in an upstairs classroom in the Academic Building, I asked my students to write impromptu paragraphs. I sat on my desk at the front of the room like I usually did. I never sat on the chair behind the desk to teach like both Mrs. Malone and Betty did. I felt the need to stand up or sit high up, make eye contact, and project to make sure I was heard. I wrote on the board a lot, and when I did that, I had to be extremely careful to keep my back straight as I lowered myself to write on the bottom of the board. This was necessitated by the mini-skirts I had started to wear.

"I want you to practice writing," I said to the class. "The more you write, the better you get, and it doesn't have to be perfect the first time. You can go back and revise and change things later. Right now, I want everyone to write a paragraph about me—your instructor—and what you think of while I'm sitting here up at the front. You get fifteen minutes. Go!"

I happened to be wearing a small neck scarf, knotted at the side. One young lady wrote in her impromptu essay, "Sitting there on her desk, Mrs. Mitchell looks like a Texian."

When I was in college, two or three of my professors had invited classes over to their houses for dinner. That seemed like a good way to get to know my students better and enhance their college experience. I particularly enjoyed my sophomore literature class that quarter; so, I asked the class if they would like to come to my house for supper. They assured me that they really would like that. On the chosen night, I was back and forth in my little kitchen preparing a big tossed salad, frying ground beef and making a meat sauce using canned tomato sauce plus tomato paste, oregano, garlic powder, and basil, and boiling a big pot of water for the spaghetti. I had sodas for us to drink. When it was all prepared, I waited. But no one came. I was disappointed, but even more than that, I was puzzled.

Some students did drop by a few other times, and each time I offered them snacks and drinks, I was told the same thing: "No, ma'am. I'll just have some water."

After a while, it occurred to me that they must have been taught not to accept food, maybe because the people they visited might not be able to spare it. I thought about Mrs. Malone and saw it was a good thing none of us took her up on her daily offer to "Ha-ve some?"

In the middle of the school year, Miss Douglas decided to move me to a very small office next to hers. I'm not sure what her reasons were, but it may have been because we were getting more new English instructors and needed space. Or it may have been because we were working together to develop a new curriculum for the BA in English. Maybe she wanted to keep an eye on me, although the door between our offices remained closed, so that probably wasn't it.

My new office was quite small, and it was adjacent to that of Mrs. Ava Jones, the English Department secretary. The plump and pretty Mrs. Jones was rather shy, very nice, and very loyal to Miss Douglas whom I sometimes heard counseling her. I now had a bookshelf of my own, a small filing cabinet, a desk, my chair, a chair for students and a waste basket.

My new office was a bit of a milestone, and I described it in my next letter to Mike. His activities in Vietnam as a Green Beret evidently were secret. When I wrote to him and my parents, I assured them that I was fine, and my teaching was going well. I'd been stressed and endured migraines before Mike went to Vietnam. Now I assumed we would resume our lives when he finally returned, and I engaged myself in my immediate surroundings and work with the students. I didn't know how the students and the relative peace in the community already were changing.

31.

Fires and Drums

B Y THE WINTER OF 1969, I gradually was becoming aware that a number of serious things were occurring on campus and also downtown. Things started happening to me as well.

The civil rights movement was the backdrop to the goings-on in all parts of black society at the time, even more than I knew. Anger erupted at odd times and places. Sit-ins and marches had taken place before I came to FVSC, made more dramatic by the assassination of Dr. King in spring 1968. Racial tensions were increasing in the U.S.

In my classes, I tried to get my students to think, not regurgitate. In more than one case, I gave a D to someone who had not mastered the skills in a class, and the student retook the class for a better grade with no apparent hard feelings. I especially remember a student from Monticello, Georgia, whom I'll call Roberta. This was after my first difficult year of teaching English majors in the upper division classes, and the English majors I taught had started to seem more generally cooperative and friendly. Roberta was an English major who had to retake one of my classes because her essays were not thorough enough, and her test average was below 70 percent. But she remained polite and pleasant in spite of having to retake the class, and she went on to a successful career as a teacher in her hometown.

Betty told me an irate husband had drawn a gun on Professor Richard Morse in his office in Peabody Hall. Not long after this, I gave a low grade to a young married woman in one of my lower division classes and asked her to come in and talk about it. Her angry husband came to my office, too. My student sat in the chair next to my desk and didn't say anything, probably because he was in the doorway behind her. The door between my office and Miss Douglas's was closed as usual, so I was on my own.

"What do you mean giving my wife a F?" demanded the husband.

I immediately thought of what had happened to Dr. Morse. But I said, "I wanted to make sure—"

He cut me off. "We paid our money for this class, and you gonna—"

Suddenly, George Washington, a college senior who had been in my class the previous year, materialized in the doorway, next to the husband.

"M' Mitchell's a good teacher!" he assured the husband. "Come on with me, and we'll have a talk."

To me and the wife who was my student, George said, "We goin' over to the College Inn."

"I'm so sorry!" my student began to say after the men had left.

"He probably doesn't understand that you can get a better grade," I responded. "Even if you don't pass the class, you can retake it. But go over what we've been doing in class, and practice writing. You can show me your practice essays. The important thing is for you to be able to write so you can do well in other classes and on your job someday."

"I will," my student said, and we began going over the essay she had submitted most recently to see where it could be improved.

This was not the last time George Washington intervened when I was in a pickle. George graduated and got a managerial position with the Georgia Power Company.

I was slow finding out what was going on in the fall of 1969 on and off the campus. In downtown Fort Valley, I noticed a doorway near the courthouse with a small sign that said "Thomas Public Library." I was upset when I learned that this library wasn't just segregated—African Americans were not even allowed to enter!

Not long after I found out about it, there was a fire in the library, and it was burned so significantly that it had to be closed. As a response to the segregation as well as to the fire, I decided to prove a point to the locals and take this opportunity to write and ask for free books from publishers. Books were sent to us, and I bought book plates and wrote in them, "Donated by Fort Valley State College." I placed these bookplates inside the front covers of the books before presenting them to Thomas Public Library. My student worker helped with this process, and later my younger brother Peter helped when he came for a visit. I hoped that this gesture would make white people in the community feel ashamed.

Eventually, a new building was constructed for the Thomas Public Library, and all were allowed to come in. But at first, blacks had to come in through a separate door, according to what was told to me by Lorraine Khoury's brother, James, a local white merchant who ran Khoury's Men's Store with his brother William at the time.

I believed my colleagues on the Fort Valley State campus who said that the students guilty of protesting and setting fires in Bishop Hall, in Ohio Hall, and in the Hubbard Education Building were only protesting the food on campus and the living conditions. However, after reviewing the campus newspapers from the times, I now realize the protests were more about civil rights.

I was caught off guard to hear drums beating in the distance on my way to get mail one afternoon. Coming closer to the student center, I saw students in dashikis and afros across the way. They were beating djembe drums in sync with poems shouted out first by one speaker and then another. Back then I knew the drums as bongos.

Words like the following may have been delivered in time to the drum beat during the protest that day:

> BE BLACK
> black, black
> strong
> from Africa we strong
> justice is ours
> be black, be strong…

Are they improvising or reciting? I wondered.

I didn't recognize anyone from my classes over there, but my neighbor David Carswell's brother Harold stood alongside the speakers. Harold looked a lot like David, but without the smile. David told me Harold was involved in the protest movement, and he used the name "Blake."

"Is that Harold Carswell?" I asked someone in the small crowd assembled there. I was sure it was, so I must have been trying to make conversation and show I was part of things.

"He's Blake," she said, "and the rhyming one is Blake Thomas. His brother is Bless."

I watched some more. I could sew, and I wondered if I could make one of those dashikis and where to get the fabric. One of the loose shirts was light tan with black and red designs in a V in front, around the neck, at the bottom of the sleeves, and around the bottom. Another one was black, and the borders were the same but in beige, black, and red.

The next time I passed the protest demonstration, I saw the education professor Dr. Robert Green with the poets and drummers. Betty told me he was like an advisor to the group. One of my African students brought me some fabric a few years later in a rich blue with light yellow and black designs around the borders, and I made my own dashiki.

Information came out about all this in the February 1970 student newspaper, the *Peachite*. The article talked about several fires, including the one that destroyed the Thomas Public Library, and the ones on campus. Eight students were arrested and released on bond. One student was found guilty, and he appealed. I knew him by sight, and I either knew or had taught several of the others.

In the same *Peachite* article, the Peach County Sheriff, Reg Mullis, was quoted as saying the fires set were not racial—which may explain why some people said the students were only complaining about the dining hall and the dorms. Mullis contradicted the state Comptroller, Jimmy Bentley, who said the students were black militants. Sheriff

Mullis said that we did not have black activists in Peach County, and that the comptroller's comments were straining relations between the college and the community.

Recently, I learned from Tommy Dortch, who was student government president in 1971, that the Georgia Bureau of Investigation interviewed students in the cafeteria and concluded that there was no threat. One of the GBI agents was a black man. It took more than fifty years for me to find out about this although the Dean of Students, Thomas Palmer, must have been aware of it then.

I continued to see the students who had been arrested. They were on campus and they were at graduation, so the crisis must have been tamped down or the accusations unproven. In front of the Education Building, the drums and poetry continued for a while.

A student editorial around this time talks about "Campus Snoops" hired due to harmful incidents on campus that presented a threat to campus security. The increasing awareness of black pride and the black power movement can be seen in articles about blackness in different issues of the *Peachite*. These were written by Bless, Johnny Jones, Willie Lockett, and Eddie Gilbert.

I didn't know, or didn't want to know, that serious activism was taking place on our campus, and I believe that not only Sherriff Mullis but also our administrators were trying to downplay it.

32.

My Veterans

A ROUND THIS TIME, I began seeing more Vietnam veterans in my classes. In the forties after World War II, Miss Douglas told me, the college's enrollment grew thanks to the GI Bill which paid for college educations for veterans. She came to the college in 1945 as that was happening, and now it was starting to happen again.

Four or five veterans were in my classes or participated in extra-curricular activities I was involved in, and I soon realized that they were not like the other freshmen and sophomores I taught. They were closer to my age since they'd done their two-year required service. And, of course, they had seen and done things the other students had not. They had gotten out of Georgia, had experienced severely disciplined training, had seen a culture completely different from any in the US, and had experienced the hazards and violence of war. They also had been in more integrated surroundings, although racism was ever present. Their service usually consisted of two phases, the first in training at a base in the US, and the second, especially for the Army, in the country of Vietnam. I think all of my veteran students had been in the Army. I don't remember any who had served in the Navy, Marine Corps or Air Force.

I did not learn about PTSD from the media or anywhere. I had heard about shell shock in relation to World I and II, but not for Vietnam. My first clue came when my student Grady Dye visited me in my office. He had been to my office before, but this time, I happened to throw an empty soda can into my metal waste basket. He reacted violently, jumping out of his chair.

"I get startled by loud noises," he said, calming himself and sitting back down. "Ever since Nam. There was gunfire and mines blowing up and bombing. I ain't got over that yet."

I knew Grady was from Tifton, more than an hour south of Peach County. He seemed stronger and more mature than most of my male students. I began to wonder if this residual reaction to being in battle had only affected him and a few others or if most of the veterans would have reacted this way.

Another veteran I'll call Wade came by to talk to me sometimes, and he shared an even more troubling story. It was about being black in the military in Vietnam. Wade was slighter of build than Grady and more carefully dressed. He wore one of those double-knit sweaters, and, because he had "good hair," a big perfect afro. I couldn't picture him in combat gear.

"Sometimes I think I'm lucky I made it out," he said. "My sergeant, he say I wasn't 'deferential' enough, so he singled me out. Made me walk point every morning."

"What is that?" I asked. I had a vague idea but wasn't clear.

"When you go single file down those jungle paths, there be land mines and snipers and traps. The one who goes first can take a fall or get shot or blown up. He didn't like me, so that was my job."

I wondered how much of Wade's natural personality had brought on that unfair treatment and how much his personality now was a result of the experience. He seemed serious, and his humor was cynical, even more so than the typical mordant black humor I had observed. Still, I sensed it would be easy to hurt his feelings.

Herman, another veteran I later met and who became important in my life, was more cheerful talking about Vietnam. But he said that when he got very sick over there, with what turned out to be malaria, his company officer and platoon officer did not believe him, so he ended up going AWOL and hitch-hiking to get to a hospital for treatment.

I talked to these veterans as well as to many other male and female students when they came by my office. I would like to have become an adviser to some student activity, but I had no idea how to bring that about, so at that time, I just continued teaching.

I had students as neighbors, including Mary, David, and Alvester. Few of the students I met on campus came to my house until later after I helped create and began advising a new student organization. One student who did make it out to visit me in the spring of 1970 was a vet I'll call Anthony.

Anthony had walked part way to my place one afternoon out of concern for appearances rather than driving his car and parking it outside. "When dudes come around to visit, they say they be 'tippin,'" he said after he came in the door and shut it behind him.

I was not so sure he was tippin' since we were just friends, but I filed the word for future reference. Like Wade, Anthony had faced discrimination in Vietnam, and he told me about it. He also told me all about his family. He and his siblings all went to or were going to college, despite growing up in a poor neighborhood in Columbus, Georgia. His mother and father both worked, but I got the impression his mother was the most involved in making sure her children stayed straight and went to school.

Anthony also had a fairly big afro, and I could tell he had some of the pride in African ancestry that was being expressed more openly among the college students now. He claimed to have ancestors from Mali and Sierra Leone.

Anthony said he was planning to work over the summer to take care of repairs for his car and save up for rent. I knew he rented an apartment near the campus.

"Are you going to stay at the Bellvue or get another apartment?" I asked.

"Nigger, you don't know what that landlord be like!" Anthony joked.

I blushed, but I didn't say anything. When he said that, I thought it showed how comfortable he was talking to me, and it seemed like a compliment.

33.

Seeing Racism

I STOPPED BY Ron's mobile home later after Anthony's visit to my place. I patted one of Ron's black cats, avoiding the kitty's dangerous claws, and waited for Ron to find his keys so we could go out to get something to eat.

"There's one male student I've been talking to a lot. He's a Vietnam vet," I mentioned. "He was at my house the other afternoon, and he told me about this neighborhood in Columbus. I think he's a good guy." Frankly, I was a little attracted to Anthony, but I wasn't going to admit that either to Ron or to myself. "He's been telling me about Vietnam, too," I said.

Ron stood up and looked very stern. We both knew my husband Mike was in Vietnam at that moment. Ron had loyally escorted me places. He taught me to drive; and we had hung out. He believed he was looking out for me in Mike's absence.

Ron already had told me about his own history of contributing to the breakup of a close friend's engagement. He thought I was about to do something very wrong, so he said, with intensity, "You better watch out! You starting to have hot pants for black man!"

I was furious with him for daring to say something like that. In the first place, I hadn't done anything although I was just a little ashamed about my feelings for the student in question. In the second place, I couldn't believe the crude attitude he showed towards seemingly any black man.

At that moment, I didn't consider Ron's personal feelings of guilt about having gotten involved with his friend's fiancé or how nobly he had tried to support me during Mike's absence. I didn't remember that he wasn't really good with words. I was just so angry and upset, I did not say anything or try to understand. When I'm that angry, my blood pressure goes up, and I literally can't speak.

This was the end of my hanging out with Ron. I didn't go by his mobile home anymore, and he didn't try to talk to me again. In the coming years, Ron would go on to become a loved member of the black community. He developed a lasting relationship with a young black woman he had mentioned to me before he and I stopped speaking. She was one of his students and had been friendly towards him. I regretted the sudden end to our talks and adventures. Thankfully, we resumed our friendship later after I returned from graduate school.

Soon after my upsetting confrontation with Ron, Anthony came by the table in the library where I was working on applications for some summer study opportunities.

As we sat there, he told me about experiences he'd had with other white folks, but I did not tell him what Ron had said to me.

"Before I went to Nam," Anthony said, "I was working at this restaurant in Atlanta. Those people watch me all the time like they think I'm about to steal something. But they all smiles." He maintained his dry, serious look. "We black folk think white people smile too much."

Of course, after that, I was self-conscious. Was I smiling too much? Eventually, I observed the kind of smile Anthony was talking about on some of the shopkeepers downtown. They wore big smiles, but the eyes didn't match.

By this time, I'd heard white townspeople, including a hardware and merchandise store owner, insult black men, not just behind their backs but also to their faces while they were working.

I walked around the corner from Main Street in Fort Valley one day and heard a store owner talking rudely to an older black man working for him.

"Get over here and do your damned job, boy!" he said.

The black man mumbled something that may have been, "Yes, suh."

I was still seething over Ron's reference to black men. I was seeing racism like this. I also was getting an inkling of what black people sometimes say about white people behind their backs. I'd already heard the black power references to honkeys and white whores. I filed all these things away to think about.

In the summer coming up, I was about to have brand new adventures, and I would learn even more about the African American experience and perspective.

34.

Rock Festival

B EFORE WE even finished spring quarter 1970 at Fort Valley State
College, anti-war demonstrations turned fatal at Kent State
University in Ohio when the governor unleashed the National Guard
on student demonstrators. In Mississippi, Jacksonville State, a black
college like Fort Valley, also experienced violent demonstrations.

Betty and I applied and were accepted to a two-week seminar at
Wayne State University in Detroit on the topic of African American
Culture and Literature. Since my family didn't live that far from
Detroit, I decided to take my cats and drive to Oshkosh first and
spend some time in Wisconsin before going to Detroit. Betty got a
flight to Detroit and a cab to Wayne State. We would have private
dorm rooms in the same dorm on campus. Back in 1965, in the small
private housing unit where my high school friend Luanna and I
roomed together in college, we'd had a big kitchen downstairs. At
Wayne State, I would actually live in a dorm and have meals in a
dining hall for the first time.

My brother Peter was finishing high school and came down to
visit me for a week or two in Georgia before we drove to Oshkosh.
I must still have been teaching classes because he busied himself
typing out the book plates for the books that publishers had donated
to the Thomas Public Library after the fire. My trailer park neighbor Alvester Burnett was nice enough to take Peter to the pool on
campus. This was Peter's first and maybe only experience in a virtually
all black environment.

When my duties were finished for the quarter, Peter and I took a
short trip to Jekyll Island, and then we headed for Oshkosh. Once

more, my limited skills as a new driver were exposed when I missed our turn-off on the expressway going around Chicago. We gave up for the day and got a motel room in Melrose Park. We opted for delivery of Chicago-style pizza and some stuffed cannelloni for supper. I asked for extra cheese on the pizza. It turned out to be unnecessary. Chicago-style pizza already has a lot of cheese, so our pizza had more cheese than crust.

I had more adventures in mind as soon as we got back to Wisconsin. First, I needed to get Pokey and Fu settled in upstairs in my parents' house with my Grandma Wallace. Emma Holt Wallace, my dad's mother, was born in a rural, Swedish-American community in Carver County, Minnesota. She grew up on a small farm, then became a schoolteacher who brought her trunk and books and roomed in the communities where she taught. Some of her students still spoke mainly Swedish. The way my grandma spoke was literate with a Swedish accent.

Pokey and Fu seemed to enjoy Grandma's place upstairs in my parents' house. Grandma had moved there after Grandpa Wallace died and the house he built in Minneapolis was sold. She still had some of her furniture as well as a floral-patterned rug that Pokey and Fu had fun with, jumping on one flower after another in the pattern.

"Oh, boy," said Grandma Wallace, watching the cats play. "Will they try to escape?"

I didn't think so, but later, Pokey did learn how to jump up and turn the old-fashioned door handles in the one-hundred-year-old house, so Grandma became very nervous and began putting chairs under the doorknobs.

All three children in my family had bedrooms upstairs there, although I was already seventeen when we moved into the house. By summer 1970, only Peter still had a room upstairs. Grandma's suite included a kitchen, living room, and bedroom, and they shared the bathroom.

I heard about a music festival, sort of like the Monterrey Pop Festival, that was to be held soon in the middle of Wisconsin. I brought this up one evening at the dining-room table with Mom and Dad and Peter. Dad was home from his office at Oshkosh State. We probably were having a traditional supper, maybe roast beef, instant mashed potatoes (my dad preferred those, saying they were "mealier"), gravy, and lima beans.

"A lot of really good music groups and bands are going to be playing at this music festival near Iola," I said. "I think I'll go and ask Jean and Jane if they want to go with me. We'll need a little tent."

Some economists my dad favored were libertarian. Socially, he was a conservative. Dad shouted at me during my senior year in high school for kissing Mike, by then my steady boyfriend, in our front hall by the stairs. Although we couldn't be seen from inside the house, Dad said he did not want me to have a bad influence on my sister who was six years younger than me.

My sister got married a few years later at age eighteen, and she and her husband took off for California, but I don't think I was to blame.

I couldn't have expected a favorable response to my idea of going to a rock festival. Mom and Dad chose the path of looking concerned but saying nothing. I was almost twenty-five years old, after all. So, I went over to Mike's mother's house to present my idea. Jane was the artist twin, and she was all in favor of the idea. Jean was less interested, and anyway she was going somewhere that weekend to get ready for community college in Illinois where she would go in the fall.

I was a Beatles fan and knew about Motown groups and, of course, jazz as well as some popular rock musicians, so I was looking forward to the music at the festival. I also thought it would be exciting and interesting to be around the hippies and anti-war types. They'd be like people I'd seen in Madison at the university.

On the day of the festival, Jane got her family's tent, we packed some water and food, and we started off. Out in the country, somewhere outside of Iola, we waited at the gate to get into the huge field already full of cars and people and the sounds of bands practicing. A local police officer kept order at the entryway, and someone took

our tickets to the festival. I drove my VW fastback through a field
where people parked their cars and set up various kinds of tents or,
in some cases, just sleeping bags and blankets.

After setting up our own tent, we wandered over nearer the
big stage. We'd brought one of our blankets with us, so we sat and
enjoyed Taj Mahal, Richie Havens, and, later, Joe Cocker, Buffy St.
Marie, and others. All around us were hippies being hippies with
their long hair and head scarves, some topless or with bikini tops,
and wearing jeans. Hippies weren't new to me since I'd been at UW
in Madison, but they were becoming more audacious. They lay out
on their blankets, some smoking joints or pipes. We had to stand
in line when we needed to use the outdoor toilet. It was all part of
the experience.

We went back to the concert area on the second day and continued
to enjoy the spectacle. But when we decided to return to our tent to
get some food, we passed too close to a motorcycle gang. The big,
black motorcycles were lined up along the path near the barn (the
only building in the big field where the festival was being held) that
the bikers had taken over and along the path leading to the stage.
In their usual head scarves, leather vests, sunglasses, and boots, the
bikers milled around their bikes watching the hippies walk back
and forth.

Although security people had been at the gate to the event, we
hadn't seen any security inside the venue. We got too close to a group
of about four bikers, and one of them grabbed Jane's arm. Jane, like
her brother Mike and twin sister Jean, was a true blonde. She was
about four years younger than me, and she had a great figure. Obvi-
ously, the bikers had picked her out with no good intent.

"Let her go!" I said sternly. I felt responsible for her safety. But
these were not men who were used to showing respect to any woman
or to taking orders from any female.

"Shut up, woman!" responded one of his buddies in a threaten-
ing voice.

I grabbed Jane's sleeve and yanked her arm away from the biker who had ahold of her. The one who had warned me away hauled off and punched me in the nose, just like in a cowboy movie or a boxing match.

I barely managed to keep my balance, but I did, which was lucky, and we scrambled away. My nose was bleeding profusely. We wound our way on foot between the hundreds of blankets and tents to my car, took down our tent, and made our way out of the huge campground parking lot. The cars and tents were packed together, so I had to turn the steering wheel this way and that to thread our way out. After we got through the gate and were headed back towards Oshkosh, I stopped by a gas station for some ice to hold on my nose. Jane couldn't drive, so I had to.

The looks on my parents' faces when we got back said what they were thinking. Many years later, I learned that those bikers had been separating couples, taking the women to the barn and raping them. They also were starting fights. Finally, the hippies rose up and fought back. One of the bikes ended up in the water tank being used for the festival-goers, and the hippies and others at the festival mostly dispersed.

When I got back to Georgia, I learned that some Fort Valley State students as well as thousands of others, black and white, had attended the Byron Rock Festival, not far from Fort Valley. I wished I could have been there just for Jimi Hendrix whom I had seen in the film about the Monterrey Pop Festival. Sadly, he died in London that fall.

35.

Black Lit and Hash

A FEW DAYS after the festival, with my nose looking better, I left my cats with Grandma Wallace and took the expressway around Chicago and the Indiana tollway heading for Detroit. The African American Culture and Literature seminar was about to begin.

I'd been to Detroit with Mike around 1967, to visit his father and his stepmother, a Detroit head librarian. At that time, few whites remained in the city, compared to the past. The Mitchells did live downtown, but on a high floor of a skyscraper with a view of the city, not in a neighborhood. By 1970 when Betty and I came to the Wayne State program, even more white flight had taken place.

I moved into my little dorm room and located Betty, who was in another room down the hall. The cafeteria was in the next building. Most of the college professors from around the country who were enrolled in the seminar being held at Wayne State were white. We all were there to increase our knowledge about black literature and learn to include more variety in our classes. When our group convened on the first day, I looked around the large room where we sat in a sort of double semi-circle as we introduced ourselves.

"I teach English at The Fort Valley State College in Georgia," Betty said, "and I am with my colleague, Mrs. Anna Mitchell. We teach literature classes and writing classes."

"Fort Valley State is a black college," I clarified when it was my turn to introduce myself. So far, it didn't look like any of the other participants were from black schools. I said, "We want to add new readings to our course outlines."

I realized that even though we were a black college, our English classes contained no African American literature. I didn't even think about African literature. I hadn't heard of Chinua Achebe and didn't find out about *Things Fall Apart* until I went back to graduate school and taught in the Institute for African American Affairs at Kent State. African epics weren't introduced to me until my Fort Valley colleague, Mrs. Jeraldine Walker, started teaching *Liyongo the Spear Lord* around 1980, and I began teaching it, too. *Son Jara* (*Sundiata*) started showing up in our Norton Anthologies later.

One of our main resources at the seminar was the paperback *Black Voices*, an anthology of African American literature edited by Abraham Chapman. "We should have Miss Douglas require this book for sophomore literature," I whispered to Betty. She nodded agreement.

The next day, we talked about our projects for the seminar. Some attendees planned to write articles or do research projects.

"Can I do an annotated bibliography?" I asked.

I wanted a project that would immediately benefit our students. I wasn't in the mindset of pursuing publication yet, but I thought maybe I could get a bibliography published.

"Give me some examples of what you'd include," the seminar leader said.

"I'd include the ones in *Black Voices*," I said, "and *Invisible Man* by Ralph Ellison, *Black Boy* and *Native Son* by Richard Wright, extra poems by Langston Hughes and Gwendolyn Brooks, a novel by Zora Neale Hurston, and the one-act play *Dutchman* by Leroi Jones in addition to poems of his."

I hadn't read anything by Zora Neale Hurston yet, but I wanted to include a female novelist. Leroi Jones, it should be added, had not yet changed his name to Amiri Baraka.

"That'll work," responded the seminar director. "Be sure to write short descriptions for the entries and include others besides those you mentioned."

Just then our poet for the day, Don L. Lee, came in to do a reading. He later changed his name to Haki Madhubuti. Like Leroi

Jones, Don Lee continued to be a star in black literature, as did Sonia Sanchez who also read to the class during our seminar. I got to see Amiri Baraka in person two times in the late 1990s, once in New York and once when he visited Fort Valley State. He seemed angry by then. Haki Madhubuti visited Fort Valley State in the late 1990s also. He worked at Wayne State by this time, and he was a very approachable individual unlike Baraka.

For our seminar class at Wayne State, Lee performed the following poem with the very strong and funky rhythm the words on paper suggest:

But He Was Cool
          or: he even stopped for green lights
super-cool
ultrablack
a tan/purple
had a beautiful shade.

he had a double-natural
that wd put the sisters to shame.
& his beads were imported sea shells
          (from some blk/country i never heard of)
he was triple-hip.

his tikis were hand carved
out of ivory
& came express from the motherland.
he would greet u in swahili
& say good-by in yoruba.
wooooooooooooo-jim he bes so cool &ill tel li gent
          cool-cool is so cool he was un-cooled by other
               niggers' cool
          cool-cool ultracool was bop-cool/ice box cool so
               cool cold cool

> *his wine didn't have to be cooled, him was air*
> *conditioned cool*
> *cool-cool/real cool made me cool—now ain't*
> *that cool*
> *cool-cool so cool him nick-named refrigerator.*

cool-cool so cool
he didn't know,
after detroit, newark, chicago &c.,
we had to hip
cool-cool/ super-cool/ real cool
that
to be black
is
to be
very-hot.

One weekend toward the end of the seminar, some members who lived in Detroit suggested a party at their house.

"We've got some hash," one of them said.

"Corned beef hash?" I asked.

Betty has never let me forget that demonstration of my naiveté and lack of cool.

We did smoke some hashish, which was significant for me mainly because my parents smoked cigarettes, and I was against inhaling foreign substances into my lungs. But I tried it, some powder in a little pipe with a little metal screen in it. If I got high, I didn't recognize the sensation. A few years later, having already done hash, I wasn't averse to trying marijuana cigarettes while trying to get a foothold in graduate studies, to see if it would help me study. I didn't have access to it more than once, though. Then I tried smoking Virginia Slims to help me focus on my reading. For me, hash was a gateway drug to tobacco cigarettes.

36.

War – What Is it Good for?

I HADN'T GOTTEN a letter from Mike after leaving Fort Valley for Oshkosh. I was nervous and excited about his R & R—his leave for rest and relaxation. I was to leave the seminar long enough to fly to Hawaii, spend three days with Mike, and fly back.

"I'm going to leave Thursday and be gone a few days because that's the only time my husband could get R & R," I explained to the director right before we sat down for that day's program.

"What is an R & R?" asked the nun who was part of our group.

"It stands for Rest and Relaxation," I explained. "He'll leave Vietnam and fly to Hawaii to meet me. Then he'll have to go back. He recently returned to Vietnam because he broke his hand in a foxhole and had to go to Japan for treatment and for it to heal."

"I hope he doesn't die in Vietnam," the nun said, with a sweet and charitable smile on her face.

I felt blood rushing to my own face, but it was due to anger, not embarrassment. Talk about insensitivity! It took effort to calm down and get my mind back on what we were there for that day.

There weren't many black people in the class besides Betty. One black lady brought out my own insensitivity, however. She certainly believed in being proper. This extended to her pronunciation of words. For her "Tuesday" was "Ti-ewes-day," and "February" was "Feb-ru-ary." The one that killed me was "Pernt," by which she meant "point." I quietly laughed at her with another seminar participant, an indication that I still didn't understand that other people's experiences have formed them and their ways of interacting with others.

Back at FVSC, I thought that Mr. McGhee's accent was funny, and I figured out that he apparently was emulating a British accent though he had not been to England. I thought Mrs Malone's "Ha-ve some?" was very funny. I thought I was laughing discretely at people who were putting on airs, but I failed to realize what caused them to feel the need to do so.

"I'll see you back at 1:30," the director said as our morning session ended.

Participants got into small groups to go to lunch. Betty preferred to go with those who ate at the cafeteria nearby. I thought it was fun to go out into the streets of Detroit, so I went with a group that usually walked to a hamburger place. It was a nice place that featured quality hamburgers with pickles, onions, Greek peppers, leaf lettuce, different dressings and cheese choices, and the usual ketchup and mustard. We always had one or two beers at lunch there. Drinking at lunch would have been shocking behavior back in Fort Valley. In fact, a lot of people didn't admit to drinking at all. It felt liberating to have our noon hamburgers with beer here in Detroit.

On the way to the restaurant, I chuckled sometimes and was appalled at other times while reading signs on windows, buildings, and even small billboards. Hand-lettered signs said things like, "Room's 4 rent," "Store Close," "Use fernitur for sell," "Liquore Store," "Julia's B Market," "Bingo play at Georg Hall." Of course, I had never lived in a big city.

Most of our seminar participants were against the war. Some of us also wanted to see the "real Detroit" when it came to music.

"I heard Edwin Starr is at the club that's near our hamburger place," one of the participants said. We all had heard his hit song, "War," so we decided to go.

That night, we got to the club and found some tables. It wasn't exactly elegant. It was dark, smokey and crowded—but still a lot nicer than that club in rural Georgia I'd gone to with Ron.

"War!—what is it good for?" Starr shouted, and we all joined in the response,

"Absolutely nothing!"

Like the club, Starr was a little rough looking. His short afro was shaggy, and he was sweating, which was understandable considering the venue and how hard he was working. Motown band members backed him up, although his record had been a solo. On TV, I had seen the choreographed steps and heard the harmonious melodies of Motown's Temptations and the Four Tops. Starr was rougher and more powerful.

The next afternoon since I wanted a swimming suit to take to Hawaii, Betty and I went shopping after class. I was still a new driver although I had covered a lot of miles by now. But I was brave enough to take my car out on the streets and expressways of Detroit. On the "Two Mile" Expressway, I was side-swiped by a black female driver in an old beat-up car when I tried to merge into a lane. I stopped my car and got out leaving Betty waiting inside. But when I looked at the other driver she appeared to be in a rage. Her car probably wasn't any more damaged than it had been before we collided. I decided to get back in my car and drive off without waiting for the police. This wasn't my first cowardly getaway, but this time my decision was based on my fearfulness of that woman who seemed a lot less friendly and courteous than the people I knew back in Fort Valley.

37.

Distance

THE FLIGHT TO meet Mike was a long one, and my first night in Honolulu was in a large room full of cots for the arriving wives of soldiers. Hawaii is a paradise, but our drab accommodations didn't show it. While he was in Japan recovering from the broken hand he hurt in a foxhole, Mike had bought me a Canon Pelix QL camera and shipped it to me in Georgia. That first night in Honolulu, I slept with it between my legs in fear it might be stolen.

The next day I finally saw Mike in the receiving area, his blonde hair short now, standing and looking for me. We hugged and kissed, and our R & R began. Getting back together in the middle of his deployment to the war was emotional.

"I got us a little apartment for a few days," he said, taking my suitcase. "It's not far. I don't think we'll need to rent a car. We can cook there and walk to the beach and look at the shops."

"Wow!" I said as we got to our rooms and stood looking out from the balcony. We weren't on the beach, but we could see the ocean since we were several floors up. Somehow, it looked more vast than from the beach on Jekyll Island even though the vista was unending in both places. On that first day, we strolled past some of the little shops where beach towels, hats, local fruits, and many pink, yellow, orange, and light green leis were on display. Then we strolled on the beach. I guess we must have eaten some supper, and we climbed back up the outside stairs to our cozy apartment.

However, we had been abstinent for a long time, and the result was that before long I began to feel the uncomfortable burning of another urinary tract infection. For the next three days, I did my best to enjoy the atmosphere and being together while I suffered the nerve-racking effects of the infection. I really couldn't get treatment for it on this short trip far from home.

"This is how the jungle looks in the rainy season," Mike said, showing me pictures he took with his new camera. "These guys are called the Hmong; they're a different people than the Vietnamese and a lot of them are in Cambodia. I'm not allowed to give out details about what the Special Forces are doing, though."

I gathered that some of his pictures could have been shot in Cambodia even though the US technically was not fighting in that country. The experiences he shared and the way he shared them felt intense. He was very focused, the way he had been during Green Beret training back at Ft. Bragg. Another feeling crept into my mind during the next few days. I hadn't been in Asia or in a war. But I had my own amazing experiences and insights from being in a new place, the South, being part of a different culture, and being a teacher for the first time. I had observed the racism we heard about up North, learned about black speech and customs, participated in the college rituals. But on the R & R, I didn't have the opportunity to share my life. It was all about the service member as I knew it should be. Still, I left feeling a little short-changed along with being weak and irritated from the infection.

We said goodbye and I flew back across the ocean, to Los Angeles, and then to Detroit. I went to the Wayne State infirmary to get a prescription for my infection. The first morning back with my fellow instructors at the institute, the leader handed me a letter that came while I was gone. It didn't have a name or return address, but when I peeked inside, I saw it was from Anthony. Not wanting to explain to Betty, I stuck the letter inside my notebook for the time being. Back in my dorm room, I pulled out Anthony's letter. It was carefully writ-ten—I was an English instructor after all—and it described how his days had been going. "I fixed my car and moved to a better unit in the apartments," he wrote. "It is real hot here. I hope where you

are is better. Well, I will talk to you when you get back to Georgia."
He didn't put his address on the envelope, so I didn't answer.

When the seminar ended, I said goodbye to Betty who took a
flight back to Georgia, and I started my long drive back to Oshkosh.

Mom and Dad were in the family room having their after-supper
coffee when I got back to Oshkosh. I wondered who was doing the
dishes since it was my chore every single night when I lived at home.

"Did you go to Hawaii and see Mike?" Mom asked. I should have
called them, it occurred to me.

"Hawaii is really nice, and Mike is doing okay. You know his hand
was broken and he was in Japan at a hospital. But now he's back in
Vietnam. I'm not sure what he's doing but some Hmong people are
working with the Army."

"We'll be glad when he gets home," Mom said. She took a quick
draw on her Chesterfield. Dad had lighted his pipe.

"I've been watching the news," Dad said. "Maybe the war will
wind down before too much longer."

I didn't want coffee and definitely not a cigarette, so I got one
of the cookies Mom made for Dad and some milk and sat on the
flowered sofa in that front room while the news was on. "I have to
be back in Fort Valley in about a week," I said. "Aunt Ruby's house
is close to the interstate highway that goes to Georgia, I-75, so I'm
going to drive to Waterville to visit her before I head down South."

I hadn't been upstairs yet to see Grandma Wallace, so I hugged my
parents good night and headed up the stairs. Grandma was watching television, too. She was a little embarrassed as I gave her a hug.
She was good at lecturing us about our health but bashful about
overt expressions of emotion. Pokey and Fu rubbed against my legs,
then Fu head-butted me as usual, and Pokey sat primly waiting to
be petted.

"I have locked the door by the back stairs," Grandma told me.
"Pokey is very smart. She can turn the doorknob now."

"I brought you some post cards from Hawaii," I said. "I wish I
could have brought some of their ripe bananas. But they wouldn't
keep, and they don't allow fruits and vegetables on the plane anyway."

"I hope Michael is doing well," Grandma said.

I told her he was and that I would have to be leaving in the morning. Then I went into my old room and went to sleep.

Leaving my parents' house and Oshkosh with the cats, I took the same toll road my family always had taken. When we lived in Wheaton, we drove from the Chicago area to Ohio every year. After we moved to Oshkosh, we drove from Wisconsin, through Chicago, to Ohio. (Little did I know that I'd be waitressing at Howard Johnson's on that same toll road in the summer of 1972 when I came to Kent, Ohio, to continue my graduate studies.)

I visited Aunt Ruby's house in Waterville, a very small town near Toledo, once each summer all my life before going off to college. Grandma Griffin, Mom's and Aunt Ruby's mother (and the mother of my two uncles and three other aunts), lived for years in a third floor apartment in Aunt Ruby and Uncle Harley's anvil-shaped plumbing supply store. Now Grandma Griffin was gone.

"I remember when all my aunts and uncles were here for Grandma's funeral," I said. "Peter and Nancy and I were here, but I don't remember if any of our cousins were."

"They were at the funeral," Aunt Ruby said from where she sat, like me, on a stool at her kitchen counter. "They mostly are older and they live around here, so they might not have stayed around after the service."

"Aunt Gladys was really emotional when she thanked Aunt Clarice for all the help she and Uncle Hutch got from her and Uncle George over the years," I remembered.

"Clarice and George got started before the Depression," Aunt Ruby said. "Your Uncle Harley and I struggled, but our store was already going then. It was harder for Gladys and Hutch and all eight of their children."

"I remember my mom and me riding in your old truck when you went around for business. I was about five," I said. "It was big, and it was hard for me to climb up in front."

"That was the old Ford truck," Aunt Ruby said.

Just then, I heard her grandson Jason yell and run into one of the bedrooms. He was after poor Pokey and Fu. Fu came out occasionally to look around while we were at Aunt Ruby's, but Pokey hid under the bed the whole time.

By the time I caught the cats and put them in their carrier so we could leave, Pokey, at least, was traumatized. Grandma Wallace she could handle, but this little boy was too much. I think Interstate 75 had been completed as far as Cincinnati by that time, and I drove down the freeway hearing growling and hissing coming from the cat carrier. When I pulled over at a rest stop to look, I saw that little Pokey had big Fu flattened against one end in fear for his life. I let him out and left her in. This meant I had to tackle the loops around Cincinnati with Mister Fu roaming the car and trying to walk under my feet while I was driving.

I made it home, but now Pokey and Fu had a strained relationship. Only a cold night could bring them to lie together again after that.

YEAR THREE:

1970–1971

38.

The Student Center Floor

M Y SUMMER ENDED with my return to Fort Valley and Buddy, the mobile home. In Georgia, it still was very hot outside, and I could smell Georgia's sweet summer growth when I rode my bike. I lived past the edge of town, and couldn't ride farther out since my road, South Macon Street, quickly turned into the Old Marshallville Road. There the pavement ended and was replaced with the reddest possible dirt both on the road and on the high banks on both sides.

I'd lost a little weight over the summer, so I was going out on my bike to keep it that way. Heading left from Stallworth's Trailer Park towards the college, I biked about a mile, then turned to go down Carver Drive past the football practice field. I felt self-conscious as usual but in a positive way. I am "big-boned" and not especially athletic, but back then I was not overweight. I was feeling good about myself until I noticed that the football team, including some of my own students, was out practicing. I didn't know if any of them were watching me and I felt embarrassed. But at least I didn't look fat.

Anthony came by to talk in a few days, and we even took a ride out on some country roads, past pecan orchards and some country churches. The windows were down (almost no one had air conditioned cars back then), and that sweet summer smell filled the car.

But right away I was focused on the beginning of the year department and faculty meetings, the usual faculty dinner, and my class preparations. I missed hanging out with Ron, and Betty was getting involved with someone new. Betty and I did go shopping a few

times. The rest of my social life consisted of going to Suzanne and
Mike Murphy's place with Clovis Tanner, the French instructor from
South Georgia who came to the college the same time as I did.

On campus, a new dining hall was being built next to the student
center. That might be what got me thinking. I'd been bothered by the
layout of the Lottie L. Lyons Student Center since the day I arrived.
Every so often in my life, beginning in high school, I have tried to
start a club or a group that would make a positive change. In my third
year at Fort Valley State College, my big new idea was that I could
help make the campus better for the students by addressing the issue
(or an issue to me) of the student center's big floor area, used only
for parties. It was my assessment that the broad expanse of floor put
students too much on display so that very few chose to walk across it.
The ones who did walk across sometimes elicited comments and cat
calls from those sitting on the side. There still were no actual chairs
or benches on the side. The students who liked to sit and watch the
world go by (as they probably did on their porches back home) still
used the cubby holes outside the bookstore as seats just like they'd
been doing on my first day on campus.

Even faculty could be embarrassed at the Lyons Student Center.
When payday arrived, paychecks were handed out from the window
of the post office on one side of the big floor. We faculty had to stand
in line to get our money, and the students laughed at us saying, "The
eagle flies tonight!"

Everyone who has gone to the University of Wisconsin in Madison remembers and loves the Rathskellar. In my time there, I would
get a bowl of chili and a drink and spend hours at a table on the
high-backed bench in one of the wood booths reading or studying
my notes or writing drafts of papers. There was a juke box and the
buzz of others' conversations, but I could work there better than in
the quiet of my room where a bed might tempt me to nap instead
of study.

Jeff and Jenny's admonition not to try to make the black college
over with ideas imported from my experience didn't connect, maybe

since I'd started thinking about the student center floor at Fort Valley beginning with my very first day. No, I thought it would be great if this student center could also be filled with booths and tables where students could sit, talk, eat, and do homework as I had done back at UW.

With this in mind, I went to see the new Dean of Students, Thomas Palmer. Dean Palmer's brother, Dr. Warren Palmer, who was a member of St. Luke's, had been head of the Education Department and, before Miss Homie Regulus, he had been head of the Hunt Library. Tom first came to FVSC as Executive Alumni Secretary. I was familiar with his predecessor as Dean of Students, Dr. Ozias Pearson, the one who told us at my first faculty meeting that *in locus parentis* was ended. Now, as the new dean, Tom Palmer supervised Ms Wellie Wilburn, Associate Dean of Women, and Mr. Wilson Gosier, Associate Dean of Men. I thought of Tom as an older person in authority. It turned out he was less than ten years older than me, and he later married someone my exact age, Barbara Holliman, a French instructor who came to the college around the same time I did. Barbara, Clovis Tanner, and I used to whisper critical remarks while sitting in the back during Division of Humanities meetings.

This day, I went across the big student center floor, climbed the stairs, and found Dean Palmer's office at the back of the suite of offices on the right side of the mezzanine floor. His secretary motioned me to go in, and I sat on a chair across from Tom, on the other side of his desk. Since his office was at the back, we couldn't see over the railing to the big floor below.

"What can I help you with today?" he asked.

"I have an idea for making the student center much better for the students," I started out. "If the school doesn't have the money, we could do a fundraiser or even use things we could get for free, like wooden telephone spools for tables. What I think would be good is to have a lot more tables and chairs, especially if they're booths, so the students can study and talk about their classes and other things in there."

I had, and still have, the unfortunate tendency to get to the point last when I talk. I also did not understand that something like bringing in rough telephone company spools would run contrary to the sense of pride the college community had in their shiny new facility.

"The student center is new, so it would be difficult to ask for more money now," Tom answered diplomatically.

He still looked friendly and encouraging, despite the doubt expressed by his words, so I continued, "Have you noticed how nobody wants to walk across that big floor? If somebody does, the ones on the side call them out and laugh."

I didn't totally understand the joking aspects of the culture (let alone the dozens—the game of insults culminating with an insult to the other person's mother). I just thought it should be obvious that this was not just a poor design but an actively bad one. "I can get some students to raise funds for some booths and chairs. Would that help?" I asked.

Tom was very non-committal. "We'll have to see."

I talked to some students about it, but nothing happened in the end. My ideal of a student center did not jibe with FVSU culture. Of course, I was never present in the evenings when the student center dances took place, sponsored by different groups, including the sororities and fraternities, or when step shows happened (synchronized dance-like movements and shouting by Greek organizations), or when pledge lines were put through their paces on that floor. It was several decades before I saw my first Greek step show competition. In 1970, I was thinking about remaking aspects of this culture to be more like mine because I thought it would help the students, and because I felt like part of the college community. I had put off thinking about whether I would still be part of this community when Mike returned.

39.

Change

I N GEORGIA and Peach County, 1970 was a turning point in several ways. Public schools were fully integrated for the first time, the 26th Amendment to the Constitution passed giving eighteen-year-olds the right to vote, and—using state and local registration procedures—college students were to be allowed to use their campus addresses and vote in local precincts, districts, senatorial contests, and presidential elections.

But 1970 was especially momentous for public school education. As Doris Bryant Booker (daughter of Henry Bryant who was principal of the black Hunt High and became Assistant Superintendent of Schools after schools were integrated) has told me, Peach County can be commended for building a new high school where black and white students would attend together. The only black student I knew of who attended the white Fort Valley High School before 1970 was Dr. Ernest Corker's son Gregory. Dr. Corker was a veterinarian who taught on campus and who had cleared a lot across the road from our mobile home in Stallworth Trailer Park to build a new house. I later learned that a daughter of Coach L.J. Lomax and his wife Mary Lucille also attended the white high school in Fort Valley, but it was explained to me that the number of blacks allowed to attend white schools under "freedom of choice" was strictly limited. The Lomaxes were members of St. Luke's where I attended, but I did not know about the lives of the parishioners back then.

Now that all public schools in Georgia were required to integrate, black and white students would learn together, except for the white children who went off to private schools.

Meanwhile on the college campus, the black pride movement was gaining momentum. For the first time, I decided to attend the coronation of the FVSU Queen during the week before Homecoming. Woodward Gymnasium was relatively new, built just before I arrived on campus two years earlier. Still, it was an ordinary gym except for the birds that came in through the windows near the ceiling and flew around daytime festivities.

When I entered on the night of the coronation, I could hardly recognize the place. The curtains drawn across the stage created a backdrop for a throne with flowers and palms and African-themed installations at the front of the gym. All the organizations' queens were lined up on one side perpendicular to the stage, and their escorts on the other side walked across to meet them, one-by-one. Each pair came to the middle of the floor as names were called. Instead of the formal gowns and tuxedos I expected, these attendants, queens and escorts wore head wraps and African print dresses in the case of the women and dashikis (with the biggest Afros they could grow and comb out) in the case of the men. Most of the women also wore Afros. John Paschal, whom I had found to be so intelligent in one of my first literature classes, wore a shirt with a leopard-skin print along with his perpetual grin.

On the day of the game, two days after the coronation, I couldn't wait to get up, drive to campus and get a place on the side of South Macon Street to stand and see the parade. Ever since those Fourth of July parades in Wheaton during my childhood, I've loved to see a parade. So, every year I went to Fort Valley State's Homecoming parade and found a spot where I could get a good view as the bands, floats, decorated cars, and other marchers went by. This day, I saw some of my students on almost every entry in the parade since English instructors teach a very large number of students. I watched the red and white Delta float, the pink and green A.K.A. float, the gold and purple float put together by the Omegas, and those of the Alphas, Kappas, Sigmas, Zetas, and non-Greek fraternities such as the Esquires. There were club floats, class floats, and the big one carrying the Homecoming Queen and her attendants.

Bands from various high schools and from whatever college we played that year were interspersed among the floats, cars, and participants who were walking. To me, the bands were the best part of the parade. Before I saw the first band, some little girls who had been practicing being majorettes walked by. They were followed by cars decorated with crepe paper, and class officers rode on top and waved.

Then the first high school band marched toward me, and time slowed as I took in the sight and realized what it meant. Black band directors walked beside black high school students playing their instruments. Only one or two of the students I saw were white. Public schools were integrated, but not the students' bands. Tears came to my eyes, and I was filled with sadness.

I happened to be standing near Diane who had been in one my classes my first year and who I remembered was from Montezuma in the next county. "Is your old high school in the parade?" I asked.

"Yeah, I went to D.F. Douglas. Macon County has a new sort of integrated public high school, but D.F. Douglas is still where most of the black kids go."

"What about Peach County?" I asked.

"They have the Peach County High School for everyone now, and there's a new black band director, Mr. Lindsey, and some white kids are in the band, I heard. But not too many came today. Most of the bands this year are from counties that still have black high schools."

A second band came by with the brass section and the drums playing loudly. It was exciting to be right next to the source of all that musical power, and the students played well though some bands played harder compositions than others. Still, even though I knew about the slow process of integration in Georgia, the parade made it feel immediate. That year and subsequent years, I fought back more tears at the parades thinking what all must be behind the seemingly innocent effort to let kids play in a band together.

I ater I learned that in the fight for equality, some college students, including SGA President Tommy Dortch, who later headed 100 Black Men of America among other endeavors, and future FVSU president Larry Rivers, who was a freshman in 1969–70, were becoming politically active. They supported Dr. Banks' campaign to become the first black County Commissioner.

Concerned black citizens were organizing to register voters and seek justice for black community members. Employees of the college, including Rev. Julius Simmons and others, met at Trinity Baptist, to plan strategies to ensure voters' rights. Hosea Williams, the well-known civil rights marcher and activist visited the campus to speak about voting.

The amendment to allow eighteen-year-olds to vote was ratified in 1970. Although only half the campus was in the city, soon students whose addresses listed Fort Valley and Peach County would be eligible to vote in local elections. That became a reality in June 1971.

Many days, I would get a coffee or a Coke in the student center and go to a table with some older students and sometimes a faculty or staff member.

"I hear the students' voting is stirring up the white folks in Fort Valley," Herbert Dennard was saying. Herbert, a military veteran, was a senior at the time. He worked for Southern Railroad and would go on to publish the *Georgia Informer*, a black newspaper in Macon.

Another veteran, Bert Bivins, worked at the Air Force base in Warner Robins and later became a Macon City Council member. Bert, who was a little more serious, said, "I don't know if they're stirred up, but a few men are filing suit against the college and the Board of Regents."

"For what?" I asked.

"You won't believe it," Herbert said. "They say it's because the school isn't integrated!"

I was speechless.

"The term they're using is 'diploma mill,'" Bert added.

Wilson Gosier, who was Associate Dean of Men, refrained from comment but had a serious expression.

"What I heard," Harvey Bannister injected, "is they want a white president." Bannister, a physical science professor, had shared juicy gossip before, like about misuse of campus supplies and facilities by college personnel in the previous administration for their own property. I knew Herbert and Bert had participated in sit-ins and maybe marches during the civil rights movement. What struck me in this conversation was the people in town calling Fort Valley State College a diploma mill. I certainly taught to college standards, and I believed my colleagues did, too. How many of the white townspeople had ever been to college?

Years later, I learned that when integration of the public schools became mandatory, efforts were made to keep black teachers out of the classroom. After strong resistance from the black teachers, that effort largely failed. Since the governor, Lester Maddox, resisted integration, students on campus protested against him. My neighbor's brother Harold—or Blake—was involved again.

During student protests, some faculty said all the students cared about was the dining hall and the dorms. That was giving the students a bad rap. But they did protest food in the dining hall more than once. Some faculty brought up these complaints at a faculty meeting one evening (we still met at 7 PM). Miss Fambro, the dining hall director, was known for keeping the students in order so I assume the faculty were used to that approach. But I had a different background, so I raised my hand.

"Mrs. Mitchell?" Dr. Banks said, calling on me.

"I want to speak for the students who have concerns about the food in the dining hall," I said when I stood up. Other faculty members bent their necks and turned their heads to look at me. "They should have more choices," I continued. "Some other colleges have salad lines and even vegetarian lines in their cafeterias these days." I was influenced both by Grandma Wallace who was a vegetarian and health enthusiast before it was popular and by my father who had carried on the healthy foods tradition and took supplements she recommended though he violated some of her rules. But now I heard that more young people, especially, were interested in diet and vegetarianism.

"We don't need to worry about that, Mrs. Mitchell," Dean Palmer responded. "The food we give them is just as good as the food they get at home."

We also debated the building of a chain link fence around the campus which happened in February 1971. I didn't stand up and assert myself on this topic, but I was against it. I thought it would cut us off from the community. But the fence was built, brick and wrought iron in front and chain link around some other parts of the campus. As a land grant institution, we had over a thousand acres, so I don't think it went all around the campus property at that time. It was done either to keep undesirable community members out or to keep students in. Given some white townspeople's attitudes toward the college, I suspected it was the latter.

Academic change was coming also. In 1970 the B.A. in English that Miss Douglas and I had been working on was approved by the faculty and went into the college catalog. The first student to graduate with a BA in English would be Moses Reginald Anderson III, from Orlando, Florida. Reggie, who was in many of my classes, was the perfect trendsetter. He was very active on campus, in sports like track and field and swimming and in clubs. But he was the epitome of laid back (or cool), responding to everything with a calm smile. He wore bright patterned shirts and sometimes bright pants—even red. But he was from Florida and refused to let the more conservative Georgia vibe slow him down. I held to my own less flamboyant but non-southern ideas also.

40.

Rap Session

I MUST HAVE been feeling more sure of myself by my third academic year in Fort Valley. I had been buying clothes at both Par-San's and Khoury's Women's Wear. Both sold good quality items. But this particular day, I went to Par-San's to look for something new to wear to work. I found a blue skirt and a top I liked on the racks inside the store and carried them to the front.

As I stood near the counter and cash register to be waited on, a college student came in. "Do you have a restroom?" she asked.

The woman behind the counter was not the owner but simply a middle-aged clerk. "We don't have none," she said. After the student left, she said to me and the others present, "We have one, but no one wants to use it behind them."

"That's wrong!" I said, feeling my face turn red and my heart beat faster. I turned and left without making the purchase, and I never went back to Par-San's. When I got home, I composed a letter to the *Peachite*, the student newspaper, describing what happened. I sent the letter to the *Fort Valley Leader Tribune* as well. I don't remember whether the editor of the *Leader Tribune* printed my letter. Based on other articles and editorials at the time concerning the potential lawsuit, I thought he was against FVSC anyway. But white people in the community heard about my letter somehow, and James Khoury says people remember it to this day. Times change, though, and people do, too. Wilton Walton who was the editor of the *Leader Tribune* back then became a community supporter of the Fort Valley State University around 2007 when Dr. Larry Rivers was the eighth president.

After my literature class one day, Michael, Jacqueline, Larry, and Red stayed behind. Michael, who always wore a suit jacket and carried a briefcase, insisted that the speaker in Langston Hughes's poem, "Theme for English B," was bitter about what it was like to be black from the South living at the Y in Harlem. We were reading this poem from Abraham Chapman's *Black Voices*, a book Betty and I used in the seminar in Detroit and that was added to our literature classes after we returned.

"No," said Jacqueline, "we're supposed to infer that he just sees himself and the white teacher as people."

"He's not that cool!" was Red's take, offered with his usual lack of seriousness.

"I'm going to ask Mrs. Mitchell," Larry decided, "in case it's on the test."

I was listening in, and I said, "We can talk about it in class tomorrow." I was impressed they were having this discussion. I added, "I've been thinking, what about having a discussion club to talk about ideas and political points of view, like about what freedom means or how we are affected by the laws of nature?"

"Sounds interesting," Larry said, and the others agreed.

"I'll ask Dean Palmer about it," I said.

A few days later, sitting across the desk from Dean Palmer again, I presented the idea. "We'd like to start a new student organization," I explained. "It would be a discussion group that meets in the evenings so students can talk about ideas, political points of view, or anything, including art and literature." In those days, new organizations did not have to be approved at a faculty meeting.

This time, Tom Palmer went along with my idea. "We can approve that," he said. "What will you call the organization?"

"They say they're rapping when they talk about things, so we can call it 'Rap Session.'"

"I'll add Rap Session to our list of student organizations," he said, writing it down. "Who are the charter members?"

Red Parker, Larry Rivers, Jacqueline Jefferson, Tommy Dortch, and Herman Holloway were the names I gave him. "We'll publicize it so there will be others," I said. "Where can we meet?"

"We don't have your booths," Tom kidded me, "but there's a nice lounge just past the elevator on the first floor here in the student center. Go down and look at it and see what you think."

"Great!" I said. "And thanks!"

Up until that time I hadn't realized there was a lounge in the student center. As he said, it was past the elevator and near the front door. Since the student center was still new, the furniture in the room also was nice and new, including gold and blue vinyl upholstered couches and chairs with coffee tables.

I had started political/philosophical discussion clubs with other students at Wheaton Community High School and Oshkosh State College, though they did not exactly take off and they ceased as soon as I transferred to other schools. But I was an assistant professor now, thinking about the best interests of my students, and I was ready to try again. I invited students from my classes to the new Rap Session along with interested faculty members.

Except Jacqueline, nearly all of the students who showed up to Rap Session were men even though I tried extra hard to talk some other women into coming. It was like the student center snack bar conversations and many other scenarios I'd experienced. The men liked to debate. The women, not so much. As a devotee of Betty Friedan's *The Feminine Mystique*, I already had a plan for raising the daughters I hoped to have some day to be independent and able to do anything a man can do. I really hoped to have young women come to Rap Session and contribute, but only a few did. Those who did, interestingly, came on their own, not as girlfriends of the males who came.

At one of the first meetings, we all piled into the lounge and found our seats, and I got out a few notes I'd prepared to get a discussion started. I thought we could discuss "consent of the governed" and see how that applied to my students' experiences and what they saw in our country. "Some people in England and France went against the idea that kings could decide what the people could do," I said, "and the people who wrote our Declaration of Independence were influenced by them. Two of those Europeans were John Locke and Jean Jacques Rousseau."

The students looked a little bored.

"So what does that mean for us?" I asked. "Do you feel like the US government is acting with your consent or the consent of your community?"

"I didn't give my consent!" joked Red. Everybody laughed.

"I guess I'm agreeing to follow the laws," said Larry, more seriously. "But some of those laws sure need to be changed! And black people didn't have freedom when our country started. Or for a long time after that. and we still have to fight to get the vote."

I was about to interject and use the Socratic method to lead the discussion a little further when an education professor I'll call Dr. Gross spoke up.

"I have brought a poem that I believe is of value to the students," Dr. Gross said. "It is called 'Our Awakening,' and I would like to take this opportunity to read it." And he did. For the next ten minutes, he used his elequtionary skills to perform rather than just read the poem he had written.

I was, as they say, fit to be tied. My dream was to give the students a place where they could argue and think about ideas—not to provide a venue for professors to build their egos. I interrupted, not very smoothly. "Thank you, Dr. Gross! Thank you so much for your contribution. Now, Thomas, what do you think of what Larry said about laws we don't agree with? Does that mean we are being governed without our consent?"

I could barely hear what the students said for a few minutes after that because I was so irked at Dr. Gross. To make matters worse, Herman, a Vietnam vet, said to me after the meeting, "I think you were a little rude to Dr. Gross when he wanted to read his poem. He's a faculty member too, and he deserves respect."

Unlike other students who came to Rap Session, Herman had decided to be an English major. He started college at Albany State, another black college in Georgia, dropped out, was drafted and went to Vietnam. So now he was in school on the GI Bill. I was amused by seeing him come to class late every time, quietly going to his seat, and sliding his somewhat tall, slim frame into his desk. He had a medium afro and big brown eyes. Though he answered questions in class, he mainly listened when he came to Rap Session.

My reaction to Dr. Gross was another case of my being culturally insensitive and wearing theoretical blinders. Southerners were more concerned about courtesy than we midwesterners were, at least at this time in our country. And, furthermore, I was a white person putting down someone older than me who held more academic degrees and who was black. I thought I knew what the students needed and wanted, as I had with the student center project, but I did not understand their traditions.

Rap Session continued, migrating soon from the lounge next to the elevator in the student center to my mobile home, a mile down the road from the campus. Fewer faculty members came when we met at my home. There, I served snacks, Cokes (various soft drinks), and beer. I think the drinking age was eighteen then, but I believed in freedom and was not extremely concerned about such laws. In fact, since I was the leader and convener, philosophies of freedom continued to be on the docket—Burke, Voltaire, Paine, Jefferson. And the students also suggested topics, including essays of Frederick Douglas. They didn't read as much as I hoped they would, but we enjoyed ourselves. I can think today of other readings we should have used, including more by Frederick Douglas and some by Olaudah Equiano, Booker T. Washington, and W.E. B. DuBois. But despite my time at the seminar in Detroit, I was only slightly familiar with those.

Considering my pride at that time in being a serious female and my love of debate, well-practiced with my dad, I'm sure I underestimated the effect these informal get-togethers with a young white female from the North—in her home—had on my male students.

It probably did help for everyone to know I was married. Fortunately, I can say that no male student made a pass at me or acted out of line. And this even in spite of the embarrassing incident when one male student (who shall not be named) came to my back door when I was still dressing, and I unintentionally opened the door before I had pulled up my jeans! Neither one of us mentioned it afterwards.

I enjoyed being with my students. And it didn't seem like there was the slightest chance during those years from 1969–1972 that I could be accepted socially in the town. My only interactions with white townspeople were in stores, banks, and the gas station. The people I socialized with when I was not in my teacher role were colleagues.

Hanging out with Suzanne and Mike Murphy along with Clovis Tanner, who was older, was like being with some of our college friends back in Madison though the Murphys were from Tennessee and Clovis was from South Georgia. Murphy was not the kind of person who criticized black students, black faculty, or black culture. He had just received his MA in Creative Writing, and this was his first job. Suzanne was from his hometown, Murfreesboro. They both seemed to enjoy life.

Before long, Suzanne and Mike found a place to rent near a lake outside of the small neighboring city of Perry. They had a big loveable golden retriever, and their home became our gathering place. My husband Mike visited there at least once after he returned from Vietnam, and Clovis came there often. Clovis was more dispirited about teaching conditions at the college or about life in general than the rest of us. He was still fun to be with, and he was courteous and kind to others on campus and off.

One day, out by the lake and before Mike returned, we were enjoying hot dogs and drinks. I was drinking beer, but Murphy preferred drinks with bourbon.

"My finger is infected," Suzanne complained. "Our dog caught a rat, and then he accidentally bit me while I was trying to take it away from him. The doctor said it's a dangerous infection. I'm taking an antibiotic, and I have to be careful to be sure it heals."

"Wow!" I said. "I've never had anything like that happen with a cat! I love dogs, too, though."

Clovis didn't even want to think about it. He just shuddered. Murphy was probably on his second drink. Maybe his third. He'd been reading Sartre and poems by Ezra Pound. He said, "Don't you know we're all going to be dead? Dead, dead, fucking dead?"

I hadn't been exposed to the F word all that long, having had a sheltered childhood. But I was being exposed to a lot of new things these days. The thought of being dead was a new one to me put that way. I was more of a romantic in my study of literature than an existentialist. At that moment, I set down my beer and looked out over this southern version of a lake and thought about it. The nun in our Detroit seminar hurt me because I avoided thinking about death, my husband Mike's or anyone's. Somehow, Murphy's words forced me to do that.

His words stayed as an irritant in my thoughts for another year or so. Eventually, I found some closure and hope, not so much from my religion as from the experience of reading Thoreau's *Walden* when I first returned to graduate school. It became clear to me after reading that book (all in one weekend) that all living things are born, go through the cycles of life, and die. We are part of nature, and it would be impossible to conceive of not being part of the cycle of life.

During my remaining time at FVSC before going away to graduate school, I sat in on Murphy's Modern American Poetry class. This is where I developed a fondness for e.e.cummings and especially William Carlos Williams and began writing poetry more seriously. One of my poems, "A Family," bears some resemblance to a WC Williams poem.

A Family

Three stones
plunk in a cold lake
clear of the lilies.

Each stone falls
away from the surface.
One ring moves

through the sky's picture,
the next begins its way,
and the third.

Three waves
peak in succession
and are fed

until clouds shiver back,
green dappled leaves shiver back,
and the blue. So

the motion back and forth
dies
and the rings are gone.

41.

Connecting with Women

M Y THIRD YEAR of teaching at FVSC was well under way.
I remained aware of Mike's imminent return but also
continued my friendship with Anthony. When Anthony told me
about his experiences growing up, it made me feel connected with
the lives of black people in surrounding Georgia towns and cities
on another level from what I experienced talking with students on
campus or even with Betty.

"My brother James is coming to Fort Valley in the fall," Anthony
mentioned one afternoon at my trailer. "Mother and Daddy couldn't
go to college. Daddy ain't even finished high school. But we all got
to go on. My sister Candace say she's going to major in home ec."

"You're in political science, right?"

"Yeah, being in Nam made me think about it. Mother wants us to
be teachers. She thinks black people can get those jobs. She cleans
people's houses."

"What about your dad?"

"Daddy, he does this and that."

I didn't push him to say any more.

"Mother makes sure we go to church, too. It's a Baptist church.
But I'm not going to church in Fort Valley."

We drank our Cokes and then Anthony said he had to go.

"I'm working at the library Thursday afternoons," he said.

After he left, I tried to picture his home and family. If it was like
many I observed in Fort Valley, they weren't as well off as I had been
even though my family was middle class and I couldn't get all the
stylish clothes most of my classmates had.

The church I continued to attend was St. Luke's Episcopal, and I even went on outings with the women I met there. With them, I heard a little about local politics and I became aware of the lives of some of the college's staff members. The ladies of the church, the ECW or Episcopal Church Women, held a bazaar every fall in the Parish Hall. A door on the right side of the nave opened to a long hallway going past the altar room or sacristy, the office, and the choir room where priests', lay readers', and acolytes' robes hung. A double door at the end of the hallway opened up to a big room called the Parish Hall.

For this fall bazaar, I came in the outside door that was at the side of the Parish Hall near the Vicarage and saw tables lined up on all sides.

"Did you bring anything?" asked Isabel Freeman. She was a member of the church who once had lived in the apartment upstairs, and she was a school teacher.

"No, I didn't think of that. I guess next time I could bring some embroidery." I did a lot of sewing, but I couldn't think of anything I could sell. *Placemats, maybe? Or cookies?*

One of the tables was stacked with aprons and pot-holders sewn by Miss Doretta Morgan. I still have one of Doretta's reversible aprons, red and white check on one side and red on the other, and one of her pot-holders. Another table was filled with wrapped pound cakes. Evidently, pound cakes were popular in the South. We had more layer cakes up North.

Behind the table that was near the swinging door to the kitchen was a big fireplace that looked like it was never used. It seemed odd to me that the wrought iron log holders on the hearth were in the shape of negro servants, sort of like the carriage boys that people used to put at the ends of their driveways. At least these weren't painted like the driveway ones. Apparently, the Episcopal donors from up North who had the building constructed in the thirties thought these were a nice southern touch. In the United States today, nearly all such ornaments are gone, and they wouldn't have been approved of even in the seventies if anyone had noticed them. But to this day, the wrought iron heads remain grinning out at the people who come and go from the parish hall. I certainly haven't mentioned them, and I don't know of anyone else who has either.

In the late fall, the ladies of St. Luke's would rent a bus and make their annual pilgrimage to Rich's Department Store in Atlanta. I had gone shopping in Atlanta a few times after I learned to drive, both with Betty and on my own. Once I bought some leather boots at a store across Peachtree Street from Rich's. The church trip included not just shopping but also lunch at the Rich's restaurant in an area on the second floor that looked out over the floor below. I had a fancy chicken sandwich that was much better than at any restaurants I was familiar with in Middle Georgia.

On the ride up and back, I talked with Mrs. Lillie Adkins, a librarian on campus who was married to Joseph Adkins, the drama professor in my department. I also chatted with Mrs. Ida Miller, wife of our registrar, Houser Miller, and with Coach Lomax's wife, Mary Lucille, who worked in the procurement office on campus. One thing they gossiped about was the recent election and the fact that our dean, Dr. W.S.M. Banks, was the first black elected official in the history of Peach County.

"I understand the people downtown are starting something to stop students voting if the laws change," Miss Ruby Parks said.

"What can they do?" I asked innocently although I already had heard something about a suit.

"It will be some legal maneuver," Miss Douglas offered. "I have heard some talk about a suit. They already have to accept the new public school integration."

"Black teachers are being threatened, I mean our jobs," Mrs. Evelyn Morse said. Her husband, Dr. Carlton Morse, taught in the college's education department, and she was a school teacher in Fort Valley.

"We will just do our jobs and trust in the Lord," said Mrs. Miller, ending the conversation.

Political and civil rights problems were not the only problems
people in Middle Georgia had, although disenfranchisement and
lack of parity surely had a spillover effect on other parts of their lives.
I soon learned a lesson about personal domestic problems experienced by a coworker.

Three of us occupied the office suite I was in. Miss Douglas had
the department head's office, Mrs. Jones had the small office leading
to Miss Douglas's office, and I had the office next to these with my
door facing away toward the interior hall. They faced the hall by the
front door. I could hear things through a door between my office and
Miss Douglas's that remained closed. Sometimes Mrs. Jones seemed
to be sharing personal information with Miss Douglas.

Mrs. Jones must have been about thirty-five. She wore business
attire: a blouse, jacket, and skirt. Her hair was straightened, and her
face was pretty, partly because of her use of make-up and partly
because her face reflected what a nice, caring person she was. In
those days, a secretary's tools included a typewriter, a telephone, and
a mimeograph machine. She made appointments and announced
visitors to Miss Douglas.

To see Miss Douglas, we entered Mrs. Jones's office first, and when
the interior door was open, we could see Miss Douglas behind her
desk, with her mixed black and gray hair, more curly than nappy,
escaping the style she'd put it in so it framed her face. She spilled
things sometimes, so I'd noticed affectionately that she often had
little stains on her dress. Her chin had a few stray whiskers. Mrs.
Jones and I certainly respected her.

One afternoon, I approached the main office door to say something when I heard Miss Douglas talking to Mrs. Jones.

"You must take care of yourself, Ava," she said. "No man is
supposed to hurt you. And he's supposed to support you, not the
other way around."

"Yes, Ma'am," said Mrs. Jones. She seemed to be wiping a tear
from her eyes.

"If you need my help, you must ask me," Miss Douglas said firmly, concluding the conversation.

Miss Douglas knew my husband was away in the war, but she didn't question me about my feelings. Just knowing how she looked out for Mrs. Jones and Mrs. Malone, the Reverend's second wife, let me know that she would be there for me if I ever needed her support. I didn't realize it then, but she probably was the one who had encouraged Dr. Palms to invite me to her home for tea during my first quarter at Fort Valley.

Miss Douglas didn't literally keep an eye on me. Since my door opened to the other hall, she couldn't see me chat after class with returning veterans, sophomore English students (often men), and the English majors, almost all of whom were women.

After the personal conversation between Miss Douglas and Mrs. Jones seemed to be over, I knocked on the door, and Miss Douglas called me into her office. We looked over the list of new courses we were seeking approval for so we could offer the Bachelor of Arts in English.

I tend to blurt out random thoughts that cross my mind, and I said, "I heard that part of Jeanes Hall is going to be used for female students." (Jeanes Hall was a men's dormitory.)

By that time, I was aware that one or two male English majors were gay and at least one or two of the male English professors as well. There also was talk about some kind of scandal. Black culture didn't seem to lean towards hiding or avoiding the subject of homosexuality, at least not compared to Illinois and Wisconsin where I had come from. And one of the apparently gay male professors was Miss Douglas's longtime friend.

That meant I was a bit taken aback by her reaction, after I had told her about a possible change in dorm populations where women would be on one side of Anna Jeanes Hall and men on the other. She said, emphatically as usual, "The way things are going around here, what they need to do is put that boys' dorm on top of the girls' dorm!"

188

42.

Trying and Failing

I N THE SPRING, Mike returned from Vietnam. I was happy to see him and resume our lives together, and he shared some of his war experiences with me. Yet having him back brought about a significant change for me since I was so involved in teaching and with spending time among students and friends.

As I've said, we didn't know much about PTSD in those days, and I don't remember thinking a great deal about what a mental and psychological challenge it was for him to leave Vietnam and the Army, not to mention the cohesive group of Green Berets, and settle down in a community and a state he knew nothing, or almost nothing, about. He did have some southern relatives, but he had never visited them here.

Mike told me how he had missed me and missed making love. I had missed him, too, but now I started to feel smothered by his affections. I went to work all day, and we socialized with the Murphys a little. However, Mike did not have a job to go to. He availed himself of employment agencies, but as an English major with no preparation to teach and no desire to do so, he was trying to stake out a plan to go into the field of communications as his dad had done. His dad had produced marketing films for Bell and Howell and Bendix.

We didn't realize that Vietnam vets were not being integrated back into the employment arena the way World War II and even Korean War veterans had been. The anti-war demonstrations across the nation had left our country conflicted, and the Vietnam veterans were not welcomed back openly, although, due to the number of southern men who had served, it may have been better in the South. After Mike struck out using local employment agencies, we flirted with the idea of moving to a halfway point between Fort Valley and Atlanta. He thought he had a better chance of getting a job in Atlanta. We even went up I-75 to the area around McDonough and looked at mobile home parks we could move Buddy to. I found myself wondering how I would be able to see my friends—including students and colleagues—if I had to commute so far every day and live in another city. Of course, in those days, McDonough was not much more than a small town.

Still trying to make an enjoyable life, we traded in my little dark green beetle for a red VW camper, and we took a few camping trips in it, including one with Mike and Suzanne who brought their tent. We camped at the Jekyll Island campground, mosquitoes and all.

But Mike Mitchell had a dream of moving to California and getting into some kind of marketing or movie production work there, and he kept thinking about that. Finally, we agreed that he would drive the camper across country to California and live in it while he looked for work there. I was to follow when the school year was over.

After he left, Rap Session met again a few times at my house. By this time, one feature of our not-so-big living room was a set of tall, expensive speakers Mike had purchased while in the service. One day, I returned home after a long day at work to find the speakers gone.

Pokey and Fu sat there looking at me wide-eyed. *They saw what happened*, I thought. *But I'll probably never know.*

I immediately called the sheriff's office since I lived in the county, not the city. The two deputies who came and looked around clearly had no idea what happened.

"When did you last see the speakers, Ma'am?" one asked.

"They were there when I left for work this morning."

"Were your doors locked?"

"I think so. Maybe I could have forgotten."

"Anyone see the speakers that might have come back and got them?"

I certainly didn't want to accuse any of my students, and I didn't think one of them would have done that. The sheriff's deputies never even asked me for the names or serial numbers of the speakers, I realized after they had left. It looked like they had no intention of furthering the investigation.

I felt horrible about the loss of Mike's speakers and even worse to think that some stranger had violated my home. I felt like I should do something, so I called one of my older students, a Vietnam vet who had attended Rap Session and who seemed mature. I poured out my story.

"I've been robbed!" I told Herman over the phone, "Do you remember those giant speakers that were in my living room? Someone broke in and stole them! The sheriff came, but I don't think they're going to do anything."

"I'll come over and see," Herman responded, and within fifteen minutes, he was there.

He couldn't do anything about the robbery, but the fact that I'd called him at this dramatic moment changed the dynamics of our relationship. I already thought he was rather charming, a tall slender man coming into my literature class late on a daily basis when he first returned from Vietnam and started attending the college. His answers in class to my questions about the readings were quite intelligent, I thought, and I've always been impressed by intelligence. I called him after the break-in because he seemed mature and smart, and I knew he was a Fort Valley resident who had been in my home. But now instead of being teacher and student, we started to feel as if we were on the same level.

I hadn't talked to Anthony much since Mike's return or after Mike left for California. We just spoke in the language lab on campus where he was a student worker. Now I started talking to Herman on a regular basis, and he would drop over some evenings to visit. He walked from his house at first, which was only about a mile. But after some dogs belonging to a homeowner who lived on the way to my house—a school principal at that—went after him and one even bit him on the leg, he started driving over in his burnt-orange Chevy Nova.

I don't think I had a clue what people on campus were saying about me at any given time, but I imagine their perceptions had changed from the time I arrived as a young new instructor married to an Army officer to the time I was hosting Rap Session and talking to more students, including male students, as friends. But there must have been talk, and this was made clear to me when the new white business instructor, a male, took me aside on the sidewalk behind the new cafeteria.

He was the one who had annoyed me earlier by congratulating me on wearing a "Ralph Abernathy raincoat." I had bought a longish denim trench coat at the Sears on Riverside in Macon because it suited my semi-hippie/semi-academic self-concept. I certainly had not been trying to imitate a noted civil rights leader.

This day, the instructor, whom I'll call Alan, wanted to intervene and put in a plea for one of his students. Phillip, as I'll call him, was a great student, very intelligent, pleasant, and interesting to talk to, and a fantastic football player, to boot. Coach Lomax used him on both offense and defense, and Phillip had grown a lot bigger and more muscular over the years I'd been having him in class thanks to his diligence in the team's weight training room. His nickname was "Crusher" due to his prowess on the field, but off the field, he was a modest, polite young man.

"I want to tell you that Phillip has feelings for you," Alan said. "He has cared about you for a long time, but he did not say anything because you were married. But now he sees that you seem to be in a relationship with another student—"

"Thank you for the information," I interrupted, feeling my face turn red. This was an unacceptable invasion of my privacy and Phillip's. "I'll keep what you said in mind," I said.

That's not what I was thinking. I was embarrassed, I felt bad for Phillip, and I thought Alan, whom I barely knew, should have minded his own business.

With this state of affairs, my third year of teaching drew to an end. However, I was in turmoil about my marriage. I loved Mike and thought he was a truly good person, but I thought I wanted my own life. I was happy spending time with Herman and doing my work in Fort Valley. I couldn't picture a new life in far off California.

I decided, or at least convinced myself that Mike was a good man but was not ever going to be mature enough to be a parent. He loved to talk about Bigfoot and other conspiracies, and he seemed to have unrealistic ideas about being a macho weight-lifter and gun enthusiast while wanting to fit into California's sophisticated communications culture. We had never even talked about having a family. He also did not understand what I had learned and experienced. Of course, I had no real way of knowing what he had learned and experienced either.

After thinking about all of this for a while, I decided to drive to California so I could do the honorable thing and tell him in person that I wanted a divorce.

43.

The Road to California

M Y TRIP FROM Georgia through Texas on the way to Los Angeles was mostly uneventful. However, it gave me a lot of time to think and grow anxious about the impending reunion with Mike.

As I drove along, I did have a radio to listen to, but it took a constant dialing for stations to find anything with both good reception and music I wanted to listen to. The motels I stayed in were not like the ones today. They were the one-story variety: just a room with a bathroom, no microwave, refrigerator or free breakfast.

Later, I wrote a poem capturing part of my journey.

Illinois Woman

*Driving alone
proceeding on through Texas
powered by a good rock station,
I swung across lanes
to a rest stop with tables,
no water or relief.
A man stood there.*

*He said, "Ma'am,
I'm from Mississippi,'
and his face lines told it,
hair grease on ends,
and sunburned sagging stomach.*

He'd been drinking, he said,
stranding his wife and kids.

They gave me water,
and honor allowed him
to take two dollars.
"Don't be driving after dark
by yourself," he said.

Back on my road from Georgia to California
I went on, hearing that man's advice to a woman alone
and "Southern Man"
playing on the radio.

El Paso sticks in my mind because there, I was almost in Mexico, and I tried chili rellenos for the first time. It was many years before any Mexican restaurants in Georgia could come close to serving food like I had in El Paso.

I thought and thought and became more anxious by the day about what I was preparing to do: to tell Mike that I did not want to be married to him anymore. One night, I called my parents from my motel and talked about how confused I felt at this point. They weren't used to getting long distance phone calls. My dad always shouted during these calls, and my mother would say in the background, "Lower your voice, Irv!"

Besides being an economist, my dad had an interest in psychology, especially William James. Dad had minored in psychology while pursuing the PhD. But, as I have said, my parents were social conservatives. My mother forbade me to date Roman Catholic boys, and my dad thought people should not kiss until they were engaged. I thought they would be against divorce. Therefore, I wasn't expecting the wise advice that my dad gave me.

"I don't think I want to stay married to Mike," I blurted out. "He is a good person, but I feel like he's never going to be mature enough to start a family. I'm not sure what I should do!"

My dad couldn't see that I was tearing up on my end of the line, not for the first time. But maybe he could hear it in my voice.

"I've been making lists of pros and cons, trying to think about what to do, but it isn't helping," I said.

"Don't try so hard to be logical," Dad said. "You need to know how you feel on a deeper level of consciousness. It would be a good idea to stop thinking back and forth about two sides of the issue and wait until your inner voice lets you know what you need to do."

I was surprised not to receive a more traditional lecture or even a reprimand, and I decided to do as he advised.

Crossing from Texas into the beginning of the desert, I stopped for gas. I must have looked like a good target to the gas station owner.

"Your shocks don't look good, lady," he said. "It's a long way across the desert, and you don't want to break down out there. We can put in new shocks for you. Won't take but an hour."

"No thank you," I said. I was still a relatively new driver, and I was a young woman alone, but that sounded fishy to me.

I finally got to Los Angeles and found Mike's small apartment. He had quit living in the Volkswagen camper after he got a job in sales. From the time I got there, we just stayed inside his place. We didn't go out to eat or to look at the sights, we just talked.

As evening came on, we lay on his small bed together, and I still didn't know what to do. I had come to tell him I wanted a divorce, but being with him physically made that much harder than I was prepared for. I wanted to end my inner turmoil, but I also realized I would hurt him, and that made me feel terrible.

"I think we should get a divorce," I finally said. "I have a life helping the students in Georgia, and you are looking for your career in California, and I don't think it's working."

He begged and pleaded with me not to divorce him, until I started to sob, and for the only time in my life, I simply could not stop crying. After a long time with me lying there sobbing and crying, Mike got so upset he resorted to violence, not against me, but by shouting and punching the wall next to the bed. That shocked me out of my catatonic state, and then I just felt exhausted.

I left the next day without making a final decision, hit the Los Angeles freeway, and started crying again, staying in a middle lane as cars passed me on both sides, hoping that I'd be able to see well enough to find my exit. Miraculously, I did, and I made it to Uncle Em and Aunt Margaret's house in Santa Ana.

Uncle Em, short for Emmett, was my dad's brother. Em had almost earned a degree in engineering, although degrees were not as important in the fifties when he got his job in California as they were later. My mom told me he had left the University of Minnesota in protest because they wanted him to take a prerequisite for a class when he already had taken and passed the higher-level class. While he was still in Minneapolis, I think, he had finally gotten married, to a Swiss citizen named Paula. Apparently, Paula was using marriage as a way to get US citizenship, and the marriage failed. He drove out to California to take a job with Underwriters Laboratories and he worked there for many years.

In California, Emmett met Margaret who already had a family but had left an unhappy marriage. Her husband was not a very kind person. By this time, when I came to visit, Uncle Em was no longer working at Underwriters Laboratories but was instead buying, renovating, and selling houses, what we today call flipping. He and Margaret lived in a mobile home that made ours look big in comparison, although they were close to the ocean, which was nice. It was an older model with a small kitchen sink. The shower also was small, so I went to wash my hair in the sink where I'd have more elbow room. I had long, straight hair I'd been growing out since my freshman year in college.

"No!" said Uncle Em. "Our hair has germs and bacteria, and you are spreading them in our kitchen!"

Margaret suffered constantly from migraines and often was sick, so they were hypervigilant about such things.

Except for that awkward moment, we enjoyed talking together. I tried to get my wits about me and prepare to return all the way across the country in my VW fastback. I adored my Uncle Em from the time I was a little girl. I thought he was funny. And I liked Margaret very much. When she died, years later, Margaret left me her amethyst, jade, and turquoise stud earrings to help me remember her by.

I was still emotionally exhausted despite having had a good visit with Uncle Em and Aunt Margaret. At this point, I called Herman on the phone at his parents' house, and I told him I wished he could fly out to California and drive back with me. I didn't think he could do it. The GI Bill was paying for his college classes, and he didn't have a job at that time. But some of his aunts helped get the money for the ticket, and he flew out to meet me.

I met him at the airport, and we started our five-thousand-mile journey back to Fort Valley.

In Texas, on a long overpass, I got pulled over by the police, not for driving above the speed limit but for driving too fast for conditions because it was very windy. I got a warning, not a ticket, and we kept going.

"You know, Georgia isn't exactly integrated," I said to Herman as we drove though Louisiana. "But I really didn't like the feeling I got from people in Alabama and especially Mississippi. Do you think it's safe for us to go through those states together?"

"Let's look at the map," Herman said.

In the end, we decided it probably wasn't safe for us to drive as an interracial couple across the deep South. We headed north and went around Mississippi and Alabama and then back down from Kentucky and Tennessee, south to Fort Valley on I-75.

I took my dad's advice. I didn't make any more charts comparing staying with Mike versus leaving him. I got back into the routine of Fort Valley. It wasn't until months later, when I was in the middle of reading *The Brothers Karamazov*, with its cast of characters from all parts and levels of Russian society, that I finally heard that inner voice. I decided on the divorce.

I didn't communicate with Mike, as far as I can remember. More than a year later I received divorce papers from him, a no-fault divorce through California courts. He initiated it because he had met someone else. Perhaps it should not have been that easy for me.

44.

George Washington to the Rescue Again

B Y THE END of the summer, Herman was staying at my mobile home a lot. I had a visit from my Oshkosh High School friend, Dorothy. Herman and I were not going out together in public in Middle Georgia, especially since he still was a student at Fort Valley State College, and I was an Assistant Professor teaching in his major.

My next door neighbor David noticed her one day while he was out washing his car. "Who is your friend?" he asked.

"Hi, David! This is Dorothy Frank. We went to high school together in Wisconsin, and we both were in Madison at the University," I said.

"Hey, Dorothy!" David said. The sounds of Isaac Hayes came from the windows of his mobile home. "Do you like that music?"

"Yes," Dorothy said quietly. Dorothy was much blonder than me and smaller than me, and her voice wasn't very strong.

"Y'all should go to my family's club in Macon, Peyton Place," David suggested. "We don't have Isaac Hayes, but there's some good music. You'll like the vibe. You can tell them that you know me!" He gave us his usual big grin.

That weekend, Dorothy and I drove to Poplar Street in Macon, parked, and went to the club. At this point we both would have been twenty-six years old, and we both would have been classified as blondes. As we sat on the tall chairs at our little table not that far from the door, holding the beers we had ordered, we were surrounded by male patrons, all black, who must have been wondering what we were doing there.

"These ladies are my friends," came a voice from behind us. It was George Washington to the rescue once again. "This my English instructor and her friend. Just leave them alone so they can enjoy their beers and the music!"

"Thank you, George," I said, as the assorted men we didn't know wandered away. "Dorothy is visiting me from Cambridge, Massachusetts. We went to school together in Wisconsin."

"M' Mitchell, she a great teacher," George told Dorothy. "You need anything while you here, you let me know!"

YEAR FOUR:

1971–1972

45.

A Modest Proposal

THE FALL OF 1971 was the start of my fourth year at Fort Valley State College. In the nation, the voting age was finally lowered to eighteen. The Supreme Court ruled that college students could register to vote using their campus addresses and that bussing was a legal method of achieving desegregation. Protesters had bombed Sterling Hall at UW-Madison, along the side of the same hill where I went to class in Bascom Hall. One physics graduate student had been killed in the bombing.

We were facing our own little turmoil on campus at Fort Valley State. At our first English Department meeting, Miss Douglas had an introduction to make.

"Faculty, I would like to introduce Dr. Sanders Walker. He is the chairman of our newly formed Division of Humanities. Dr. Walker's wife, Dr. Emma Walker, has already been with the college as Director of Remedial Studies. The other departments making up our division include Music, Art, and French, which will now be called Foreign Languages."

We looked at each other.

Dr. Walker stood to the side with one leg crossed in front of the other as if he were posing for a magazine cover.

He said, "It is a great pleasure to join your institution and to be given the honor to lead such illustrious department heads and faculty." He turned to Miss Douglas. "Please do not omit the inclusion of Spanish, speech and philosophy classes within our new division, Miss Douglas."

Miss Douglas smacked her lips together. We wondered what she
was thinking, but all she said was, "That is certainly true, Dr. Walker.
Please excuse my omission."

"All faculty in the division are invited to a luncheon to inaugurate
our new leadership structure," he continued. "I have decided to give
our inaugural luncheon the title, 'A Modest Proposal,' as I will be
laying out the plans for our new division. We will meet in the large
room on the second floor of Peabody Trades Building, which is the
building housing my new offices."

Dr. Walker was a very light-skinned African American, white-
haired with a white moustache, very slim, of medium height, and
very dapper in his choice of shirt, tie, jacket, and slacks. His clothing
was light-colored, like what I pictured a southern colonel would
wear—like Col. Sanders.

After the meeting, when Dr. Walker and Miss Douglas no longer
were in the room, we all started talking.

"Miss Douglas has been here since 1945," said Doris Adams. "How
can he credibly tell her what to do?"

"Because he's *Dr.* Walker," someone suggested.

"Mr. Mathis and Dr. Hicks have led their programs for a long
time, too. Why do we need another layer of administration?" Mike
Murphy wondered.

JC agreed. Betty and some of the others didn't say anything, but
they looked unhappy about the situation.

I couldn't help blurting out what I had been holding back. "'A
Modest Proposal'? For a luncheon?"

Some of the other English instructors laughed.

"That's the title of the satire by Jonathan Swift in which he
proposes eating babies," I said, "—a satire against the English allow-
ing poverty to continue to exist in Ireland!"

It wasn't a good start. We preferred our department heads even
if we didn't always agree with them. They were almost like parents.
Well, Dr. Dallis, who was over the Art Department, was a little
younger than the other department heads, but he was a very big

man with the presence that can go along with that, so he was very respected, too. He had been trying to get art recognized as a major, and at least one of my students, Archie Muckle, Jr., wanted to change his major to art. I wondered how this new Division of Humanities was going to affect that process.

Later that day, I found out that my class schedule was being changed, but it could have been worse. Miss Douglas called me into her office.

"We are doing a self-study in preparation for reaccreditation," she said. "Now that schools are becoming more integrated, the Southern Association of Colleges and Schools might not give us such easy approval as in the past. You have asked to teach an extra literature course each quarter," she continued, "and I've been able to let you teach Shakespeare, Eighteenth Century British, and the Victorian Novel. But I can't do that anymore because we can be criticized if they see that faculty regularly teach overloads."

"I understand," I responded. It had been interesting while it lasted teaching these literary periods and authors.

"Dr. Walker has asked to teach the Survey of British Literature classes, but I told him I was happy with the job you have been doing, and I would prefer not to make that change," she told me.

So far, Dr. Walker and this new level of administration were not making a good impression on me. How could he sweep in and tell Miss Douglas how to assign the classes in a department she had been head of for years — certainly before I came on board? I was a little angry, but not as angry as I would have been if my survey classes had been taken away. I thought I was finally succeeding with the English majors and giving them a good foundation in the literature of the British Isles.

Miss Douglas moved some papers on her desk and said, "Now that our BA in English has been approved — thanks to your hard work — we can begin advising students. We don't have to start with freshmen. Students who are beginning their junior year are eligible to change to the new major. Who do you have in mind?"

I smiled. I always smiled when I thought of Moses Reginald Anderson, III, or Reggie.

"You know, I've already talked about it with Reggie Anderson," I said, "and he wants to change his major."

"There's one more problem," Miss Douglas said. "It is too late for a student to register in remedial classes, and anyway they are zero-credit classes. One of our male students needs three more credits. You know he could be drafted if he is not taking enough hours in school. I have agreed to let him register for the introductory freshman English class even though he is supposed to be in remedial English. I know you are sensitive to this issue. Would you be willing to work with him outside of class if I put him in your section?"

Of course, I said yes. And that is how I met Lucius Dodd. Since then, he has gone on to be an insurance agent and then owner of his own printing company in Atlanta. It is a pleasure to see him when he returns for Homecoming, and we both stand near the front of the campus to watch the parade. I see him at football games, as well.

That fall of 1971, Lucius came to see me in my little office after all the registration issues were handled.

"Hello, I'm Mrs. Mitchell," I said.

Lucius said, "Yes, Ma'am," and he shook my hand.

He was very polite and very reticent. When I picture his face, I seem to remember that he had eyes that are lighter than ordinary. When he came to my office, we worked on verb forms, sentence structure, and paragraphs. He had assignments to do.

"What is the answer to number seven?" I asked after he sat down at the next meeting.

He looked at me with those eyes but couldn't bring himself to say anything although it looked like he had written an answer on the paper.

"Is it 'lie, lay, lay'?" I asked.

He nodded silently.

And that is how most of the sessions went. Lucius passed English 101, signed up for my English 102, and continued coming in for extra tutoring the next quarter. Looking at his success in life, I'd say college worked for him, and he worked to make it happen.

Our new Division of Humanities was a disruption on campus, and disruptions continued in the community as well. When I went over to the larger faculty office and talked with JC, he told me he was concerned about the goings on in the country, in Peach County, and on campus, shaking his head to comment as he always did.

"They'll be bussing the children in Peach County, the Supreme Court says," JC mentioned.

"I think one of my students, Larry Rivers, is working with the people registering students to vote," I said. "I thought of that because he's from Pennsylvania, and his friend, Mark Davidson is from Pennsylvania, too. Mark wrote an essay for my class about being bussed in from the city to a school in the suburbs and being shouted at and called names as the bus went past white protesters."

"That's how it be," JC responded, shaking his head. "These college students got the vote now, and Georgia probably can't keep them from registering to vote here. Have you been hearing about that suit?"

"I heard a little from the church ladies."

"Some town folks, a father and son, are doing it. They say we're a 'diploma mill.' They're wanting a white president for Fort Valley State College." He shook his head again. "Some of the white faculty lining up with them. Have you seen that chemistry professor who wears the cowboy boots and hat?"

I'd seen him, but I couldn't remember his name. I was just feeling sad. It was selfish, but I had loved becoming part of my department and my school and even my church. I was part of a little community with my trailer park neighbors. We had at least one white student on campus, Connie Copeland. She didn't have any problems fitting in as far as I could see. Others surely would be welcome. I wondered again how many white people in town even had a college degree besides the teachers, doctors, and lawyers.

46.

Older but not Much Wiser

I T WAS TIME for me to start thinking about my future.
My personal life had certainly changed. Mike was still in California, and I was still in Georgia. I had fulfilled the recommendation of the Wisconsin graduate director Standish Henning that one should teach for a while before going on to pursue the PhD. My classes were going very well. The wonderful thing about teaching literature, writing, and logic is that we continue to learn, perfect our skills, and get a better understanding of things as we teach.

In college, I had taken at least two English Romanticism classes plus a survey that included Wordsworth, Coleridge, Shelley, Byron, and Keats. Among these poets, I had never cared much for Percy Bysshe Shelley. By teaching his work in my own classes, especially "Ode to the West Wind," and "Prometheus Unbound," I began to understand and appreciate the poems myself. "Ode to the West Wind," is a beautiful expression of how life is part of nature and a consolation for the shortness and incompleteness of human lives. I can still read it in the textbook we used for British Literature Survey in the classes I taught, complete with my lecture notes written between the lines. "Prometheus Unbound" finally came alive to me when I taught the students how to analyze its structure.

So, it was time to follow in my dad's footsteps again and get the PhD. I took the obvious next step and started looking into applying for graduate schools.

Herman came by my place quite a bit now in his orange Chevy Nova.

"I'm applying to about ten graduate schools," I said as we sat in my kitchen. "I think the colleges in Ohio are good, so I'm applying to Ohio State, Bowling Green, and Kent State. Did you know I was born in Ohio?"

"Whoa," Herman responded. "Isn't Kent State where the students got shot?"

"Yes," I said, "but I think it's really a more normal place. They don't have as much protesting as Madison, where I got my BA and my master's. Their governor just went crazy and called the National Guard—who also went crazy. Anyway, the scores from my GRE are still good—that's the exam you have to take to get into graduate school; and I'm waiting for them to send my scores to the grad schools I'm applying to."

Herman liked creating things. "I'm finishing up writing this play, and Melvin Freeman and Jimmy Little are going to play parts in it," he said while sitting at the card table I used for a kitchen table.

Herman was in Mr. Adkins's drama class as part of his studies as an English major, and the Fort Valley Players were going to put on his play in the Academic Building auditorium. He was in the English Club, too, which was required. He was supposed to work on either the *Peachite* or the *Flame* yearbook, as well, but hadn't started either of those experiences yet. He wasn't taking any of my classes at the moment, which was just as well, because I didn't want all those female English majors to suspect that we were seeing each other. Looking back, I'm sure there was nothing secret about it.

We had gone up to Atlanta a few times, including to Piedmont Park. There seemed to be hippies hanging out there. But mainly, we sat around my place and talked.

It seemed like life was getting more complicated as I finished my fourth year of teaching. That fall, I had taken on a part-time job teaching in Upward Bound, a federal program for high school students to help prepare them for college and provide enriching cultural experiences. Our Upward Bound classes met on Saturday mornings. Mrs. Gladys Toomer and I taught the English classes. John Dubriel and Freddie Riggins taught the math. Mrs. Allene Lawson taught speech, although she herself had serious hearing problems. Mrs. Lawson was quite confident and outspoken. There were a few other faculty members, as well, for electives like art and social science. John Taylor was the director. Taylor was a young man whose wife worked on campus in the administration. Mrs. Ida Miller, from my church, was the counselor.

I had one Upward Bound female student I remember as Veronica, who I thought was particularly beautiful for a high school student. She was shy like most of the others. To give an idea of how many connections can exist in a small town, she is now married to the real estate agent who handled the sale of Herman's grandmother's cousin's property to us out on the same road where Stallworth's Trailer Park was. We live in that house now. In the seventies, the road was called the Old Marshallville Road, but now it is part of State University Drive, and it is paved.

On one of these Saturdays early in the year, I was asked to make a run from the Miller Science Building where we held our classes back to another building to get some teaching supplies stored in a cabinet there. That building, Hubbard Education, was on an incline. The front door was on the second floor and stairs went down to the first floor that also had a door on the ground floor at the side. I went down the steps to the first floor of classrooms, went in the first one on the left, and opened one of the cabinets on the wall below the windows. As I looked inside, I felt a pressure on my back, and I looked sideways to see an older man I'll call Dr. Finton. He was pushing himself up against me.

He pinned me against the cabinet, but I said, "Stop!" in a loud voice and twisted away from him. He reached for me, but I grabbed the supplies and ran up the stairs and out of the building.

I couldn't believe what had just happened. I stopped to breathe outside the building before I went back in my Upward Bound class. I didn't report him. I didn't say anything, although I have recounted the story in the years since. I was just glad at the time that I got away.

I kept teaching my freshman, sophomore, and upper-class English classes and going to all the meetings. I confess that at Dr. Sanders

Walker's meetings, Barbara Hollimon, Clovis Tanner, and I sat at
the back and muttered critical remarks and jokes.

"He's reading us his obituary again," whispered Clovis as Dr.
Walker announced that he had just received some kind of recognition and began summarizing his entire career.

Barbara chuckled. She had been a student of her department
head, Dr. Hicks, and she didn't appreciate how Dr. Walker now
overshadowed her mentor.

"Don't forget our tea in the Cathedral in the Pines," I injected.

That had been a social event at his modest ranch style home on
South Macon Street just past the college, where we sat on folding
chairs under the back-yard pine trees and had one cookie and a cup
of tea.

Once again, I was guilty of ridiculing someone without taking his
contributing life experiences into account. But under Barbara's and
Clovis's influence, I had help.

Mardi Gras time approached, and this meant the Alumni Kappas
began selling tickets for the Kappa Mardi Gras dance, to be held
in the Macon Auditorium. Since it was a fundraiser, and buying a
ticket equaled a vote for one of the ladies running for Queen of the
Mardi Gras dance, they needed participants. Dr. Dubriel asked if I
would be willing to be one of the candidates for queen of the dance.
My Betty Friedan side didn't like the idea. In fact, I'd always disliked
overly feminine displays — like shrieking at bugs — and held a bias
against the girls who ran to be queens of this or that. But it was a
fundraiser, and in all honesty, I was pleased to be asked to be more
a part of the community, so I agreed.

Two other people running were Ms Eva Adams, a history instructor the same age as me, and Mrs. Otis Redding, wife of the famous
deceased Macon rock and roll and blues singer. I really was impressed
to think I would meet Mrs. Redding. Soon after I had come to
Georgia, Otis Redding had died in a plane crash in a lake close to
the Madison, Wisconsin, apartment Mike and I lived in there. I had
seen Otis Redding, along with Jimi Hendrix, in the movie about the

Monterey Pop Festival. I felt honored to be part of something Mrs. Redding was in.

The trouble was that I needed a date or escort.

Herman sat at the table in my kitchen one afternoon. He was sketching something while I tried to figure out what had happened to my request for my GRE scores to be sent to several graduate schools. They reported that they had not received them.

"I think I've missed the deadlines to get into these programs because they didn't get my scores," I complained. "I don't understand what went wrong. GRE has my scores on record from 1967, and they're still good."

Herman stayed busy with what he was doing. "Can you get permission to submit a late application?" he asked.

"Kent State at least told me about the problem. I think I'll resend my scores there. I'll write a letter asking for a teaching fellowship and describing my experiences."

"By the way," I added. "I agreed to run for Mardi Gras queen for the Alumni Kappa. It's a fundraiser. I've never done anything like that, but I guess it will be an experience."

"You'll do great," Herman encouraged.

"I have to have an escort, though, and since you're still a student and an English major, and I'm an English instructor, it won't work for you to be my escort. I'm thinking about asking James Timley. He's from Macon. He was in graduate school with David Carswell. Some of those Macon people I talk to at the student center, Herbert Dennard and Bert Bivins, are friends of his. That's how I know him. Timley is teaching in a middle school in Macon."

"I guess that's OK," Herman said.

"What are you working on over there?" I asked.

He picked up the piece of paper and showed me. It was a sketch of me.

"You're good at drawing!" I said, blushing. "I wish I was. I can draw houses and flowers, but I just can't get it right when I try to draw people's faces or even animals. They always end up looking like something else, not what I was trying to draw."

The tickets for Mardi Gras had been sold, but the winner would not be announced until the night of the dance at the Macon Auditorium. I had sewed a dress for myself. I still resisted the whole Miss America or homecoming queen stereotype, so I made a long dress out of a dark knit fabric that had an ethnic-looking repetitive pattern in navy, white and dark pink and a border around the bottom of the skirt.

The part I dreaded was the actual dancing, but when we got to the auditorium and out on the floor, I could tell that Timley was good at leading. I just tried hard to remember how to do the two-step. I thought to myself that he'd probably be a superb dancer if he had a different partner.

The auditorium decorations looked very elegant, containing a lot of red and white since those are the Kappa colors, but I thought it was strange for such an elegant occasion that the guests had to bring their own liquor just like at that club I had gone to with Ron.

The time came for the crowning of the winner, and we contestants stood in a row on the stage. *I do not know how to do a Miss American smile,* I thought to myself. I blushed, and put on the biggest grin ever, feeling like the Cheshire cat. In the end, Mrs. Redding was the winner, I was first runner-up, and Ms. Adams was second runner-up. That was my first and last experience being a pageant contestant, but at least I have a story to tell. The dance was very formal and impressive except for the part about BYOB.

I was handling my job, my extra job, and my social life. Only a few more events lay between the Mardi Gras dance and the end of the third quarter of my fourth year at Fort Valley State College.

47.

Mrs. Ida Miller

I T WAS TIME for us to take our Upward Bounders on their big
cultural field trip for the year. We were going by bus to Atlanta to
hear the symphony and to stay overnight at the well-known black-
owned hotel, Paschal's. This establishment also had a fine restaurant
and musical entertainment in its lounge on some evenings. I really
was hoping for jazz.

Interstate 75 had just been completed between Peach County and
Atlanta, so the bus full of high school students, teachers, and the
Upward Bound counselor drove smoothly up the uninterrupted two
lanes going north. I felt fortunate when I was joined on my seat on
the bus by the counselor, Mrs. Miller.

I already knew her a little from going to St. Luke's and going on
the Episcopal Church Women's trip to Rich's the previous year. Mrs.
Miller was from Atlanta originally, not from a small town. She and
her family—her husband and three children—had lived for a while
in New Orleans while Houser Miller worked at Dillard University.
He had grown up in Crawford County, just north of Peach County,
and his father, James Isaac Miller, was one of the founders of Fort
Valley State, originally Fort Valley High and Industrial School.

"I hope the students appreciate and enjoy the symphony at the
Fox," Mrs. Miller said.

"I haven't been to many live orchestra performances," I said. "But
I like to listen to Baroque music, especially Bach, and to Mozart.
Maybe I'd enjoy more musical periods better if I hadn't stopped in
the middle of auditing that music appreciation class in college."

"We'll see how they like it," said Mrs. Miller. "But at least they will have had their first exposure to it."

"Oh, look at the beautiful dogwoods in bloom!" she exclaimed suddenly.

Along the edges of the woods, we passed on the expressway, slender trees were in bloom with their floating white flowers.

"Have you noticed how the blossoms seem to face up to the sky—or to heaven—instead of poking out in all directions? I believe dogwoods will always be my favorite trees," Mrs. Miller said.

It wasn't just what she said, but how she said it. To this day, I think of Mrs. Miller with joy every year as I seek out the dogwoods, the ones in the wooded areas, not the rounded ones planted in yards that don't convey the same sense of layers of floating blossoms.

We arrived in downtown Atlanta, and after our bus driver parked, we herded our students through the front doors of the Fox Theater. It was the first time I had been there, and I thought it was majestic. The only other large city theater I had been in was in Chicago where I saw *Oklahoma* performed. I was a teenager then myself.

The students visited the restroom, and then we guided them to their seats. For a while, the students looked impressed, but part way into the actual symphony performance, they became restive. We had to shush them as they started to talk. It was true that they were being exposed to culture, but they did not have the background or context to enjoy it very much. They probably had played in bands, but not orchestras, and some of them were going to take a music appreciation class as part of their future college curriculum, but not all.

After the performance was over, we got back on the bus and drove a little way west in Atlanta to Paschal's, near the Atlanta University Center where Atlanta University, Clark College, Morehouse College, Spelman College, and Morris Brown College—all private black higher education institutions—are located. Not long before, African Americans were denied entry to white hotels and restaurants, so Paschal's was a mecca and a tradition for blacks.

The students were shown to their rooms first, and soon we all met in the restaurant. We ordered from a menu and were served at our tables. Our Upward Bound faculty and staff guided and assisted the students. I think most of the students chose fried chicken, and I probably did, too. There was a small jazz band preparing to play, but our charges were high school students, and we didn't want them staying late in the lounge where alcohol would be served, so they went to their rooms after they had eaten. At least there were several to a room so they could socialize there before going to sleep.

Most of the adults returned to the lounge downstairs to enjoy the jazz and a drink. It was part of my mission in life to hear live jazz, so I was very happy to be here. As I sat at one of the tables, one of the male instructors, I'll call him Marvin, came up and sat with me. I had chatted with Marvin at faculty meetings a few times, and I also knew his wife.

After about thirty minutes, Marvin said, "How about joining me in my room? Come on, we're out of the Valley—why not?"

He should have realized I knew he was married. Maybe he thought I was single now since my husband had been away for so long. He didn't know my business, I don't think, and I wouldn't have been interested in him anyway. I shook my head no.

"Come on, I had a special friend back in South Carolina, and she was white. It didn't cause any trouble," he said.

"No, thank you!" I said, wondering if this was the normal thing to say in the situation. "I'm going back to my room now. Good night!"

I got to know Mrs. Miller a little more on the trip back. I learned that her older children Isaac and Rhoda had grown up mainly in Louisiana and were nostalgic about it. Elizabeth, the youngest, had grown up more in Fort Valley. The family had moved back to Mr. Miller's ancestral home in Crawford County, just outside of Fort Valley. It was a two-story farmhouse. Some other Millers and relations had lost their land out there for non-payment of taxes levied by the white city and county governments. Ida and Houser's children put themselves through college with money from selling their peaches at the road in front of their house.

A little while after we got back, Mrs. Miller invited me to that house for dinner. To me, the Miller home was the ideal of what educated humanists should strive for, and as a student of literature, I considered myself a humanist. It was not fancy and had not been the subject of professional interior decorating, but the chairs and sofas were of good quality, and the dining table was solid, good quality wood. Shelves of books and art objects lined the walls. Colored glass bottles were arranged on the high windowsill near the dining-room table.

As soon as I got a home of my own, I created a place for colored glass bottles and glasses and little pitchers. There are red, blue, purple, green and yellow colored bottles, glasses, and pitchers in my kitchen window today. As with the dogwoods, I think of Mrs. Miller when I look at them.

48.

The Next Phase

"I GOT ACCEPTED to Kent!" I told Herman when he came in the door. He had been at his mother and father's house where he usually stayed when he wasn't in classes, doing things with his friends (like practicing a Four Tops routine with his friend Chico), or coming by my house.

"And they have offered me a fellowship to teach two classes every semester. They don't have quarters, just two sessions a year plus summer school. I'm waiting to see if I get that federal stipend through Fort Valley State. Then we'll have enough money to move and take the mobile home with us."

"Okay," Herman said. "I'll apply to Kent, too, and see if I can transfer. My grades are better."

Now, after serving two years in the Army, he was doing well at Fort Valley State College, and the GI Bill helped to pay for his tuition. We waited to see if he'd get accepted at Kent, too.

Herman and I were not being open about our relationship, but evidently the word had spread. One day he told me that his mother had been approached by the daughter of one of my English colleagues who was a member of St. Luke's. Herman's mother had been confirmed at St. Luke's when she first came to Fort Valley, and Herman had attended Sunday School at St. Luke's. Now his mother was a member of a different church, Usher's Temple CME.

The young woman who had spoken to Herman's mother was close to my age and seemed a little reserved but friendly the few times I had met her. She attended college in another state. Apparently, she had heard that Herman and I were in a relationship. According to Herman's mother, the young woman, I'll call her Judith, had visited Herman's house to give his mother a warning.

Herman said, "Mother says Judith came to the house yesterday to talk about us. She told her you are no good for me, and I need to end my relationship with you so I don't get hurt."

"I barely know Judith!" I said. "Are her family and your family close?"

"Not really," he said. "My parents are schoolteachers. The college faculty know all the teachers in town, but the two groups don't socialize much unless they're members of the same church. Kids go to school together, so they're more likely to play together. But the teachers and college folk don't really socialize that much."

Herman's parents both were teachers. His father had worked previously as a building and grounds manager on campus, and at one point the Holloways had their own café frequented by college faculty and students. Mr. Holloway taught history and social science in the public schools. Herman's mother taught kindergarten. She had done her part in a protest so black teachers could keep their jobs, which had been threatened after integration.

"Don't worry about it," Herman said. "Mother didn't seem like she was trying to make me do anything. I guess she just wanted me to think about it. And she does like controversies and issues!"

Herman hung out a few times with a faculty kid he'd gone to high school with in Fort Valley. Herman had used marijuana and hash in Vietnam, so he wasn't averse to getting a little high. But this faculty member's son had offered him a drug that gave him a bad trip. Maybe it was speed or LSD. The night it happened, Herman came by my place feeling terrible, and I worried about him until his reactions finally slowed down and diminished.

Herman also hung out with Mike Anderson and brought him over to meet me once. Mike Anderson was the interracial son of Canadian parents, and he had journeyed all the way to Fort Valley to attend the Byron Rock Festival—and I guess to see what black culture in the

South was like. He crashed at different college students' apartments and was harassed by the local police. I can picture him with his big, light brown afro and tight-fitting shirts. He was the first interracial individual I met, at least to know it. We didn't know that we would have our own interracial sons one day.

The people I socialized with the most at this time were the Murphys, and I introduced Herman to them. One evening we drove to Perry and had some food and drinks at the Murphys' home by the lake. They knew Mike, and I wanted to be up front with them about my new relationship and have Herman meet them. It seemed like a pleasant evening with no problems.

But Mike Murphy dropped by my office the next Monday and expressed a sentiment that was not as harsh, but in a way similar, to what Judith had said to Mrs. Holloway.

"I think Herman is a very nice person," Murphy started out. "And we enjoyed having you all over. What are your plans for the future, especially since you're going to graduate school in Ohio next year?"

"Herman just got accepted at Kent as a transfer student. He'll be an English major in the undergraduate program," I said. "We're going up there together and moving my mobile home up to live in."

"I don't think you'll be happy if you end up getting married," Murphy said. "After a while, you'll begin to realize that you do not have enough in common."

I didn't argue with him, but I didn't think it was his business, and I didn't consider taking his advice. I felt angry with Judith and disappointed in Murphy and Suzanne. But their opinions reflected the cultural attitudes of the majority of both black and white people in those days and for a long time after.

"It's going to take my whole summer stipend to pay for moving the mobile home to Ohio," I told Herman. "Are you going to drive your car separately, or can we get a hitch and haul it?"

Since my car was smaller than his, we got a hitch for his car, and pulled mine. Just like Mike and I had chosen a site for Buddy sight unseen in Georgia, Herman and I chose one in a trailer park called Apple Orchard in Ravenna, Ohio, near Kent, for Buddy to be delivered to.

We put the cats in carriers (two separate ones since my trip from Ohio a few years earlier had damaged Pokey and Fu's relationship), and we set off for our new school. The move did use up my first available funds, so I didn't enroll in summer school after we got there. However, I sat in on a class in American Transcendentalism, and the professor, Dr. Sanford Marovitz, offered to let me register later and get credit for the class if I did the work that summer. Dr. Marovitz later was very helpful as the first reader on my dissertation. Catching up in the American Transcendentalism class that summer is how I came to read all of Thoreau's *Walden* in one weekend.

During fall semester, after we developed friendships with many English graduate students, Herman had an attack after drinking some beer. A cystoscopy was done, sending a little camera up to Herman's kidney. Herman said he had very weird dreams while that procedure was taking place. The cystoscopy showed that one of the kidneys was no longer functioning most of the time. Our doctor decided his kidney should be removed.

Herman was intolerant of anesthesia, and his heart stopped during that operation. Doctors had to hurriedly finish the operation in order to restart his heart. His recuperation took a few days in the hospital because they had to be careful he didn't get an infection after they turned him over to restart his heart. That traumatic crisis undoubtedly helped cement our relationship.

In the next three years at Kent State, I completed my PhD coursework, passed my written comprehensive exams, taught in the Institute for African American Studies, taught the English department's minority literature class, got my dissertation topic approved, and completed the first chapter of my dissertation.

While we were in Ohio, in January 1973, I received a final notice of my divorce. In July of that year, Herman and I got married with Debbie and Lawren, fellow graduate students, as matron of honor and best man. In the beginning of the summer of 1975 before our return to Fort Valley State College, our first son, Aaron, was born. When he was three months old, we left Buddy behind. We returned to Fort Valley, and we moved into one of the new faculty apartments.

Epilogue

W HEN HERMAN, AARON, AND I got back, I heard that Dr.
Sanders Walker said, "She went for a PhD and came back
with a baby."

Be that as it may, I continued to teach in the English Department
at Fort Valley State College, now University, for a total of forty-six
years. I finished my dissertation in 1979, right before our second son,
Alexander, was born; and I defended it successfully that fall.

At the time of our return in 1975, Georgia was about ready to cele-
brate the Bicentennial. According to research I did later as a faculty
intern on the *Macon Telegraph*, Fourth of July celebrations in most
Georgia towns had been limited to picnics for the white people and
concerts by popular musicians for the black people. But beginning
in 1975 and lasting for several years, Fort Valley had fireworks shows
at South Peach Park, the fairly new county park that welcomed all.

We stayed in the faculty apartment on campus until Aaron was
three, and then we bought a small country house built on ten acres
of land that was half woods and half field in nearby Macon County.
We looked around at different properties before deciding on this one,
owned by one of my students, Jackie, a white male English major,
possibly the first as well as the last white male English major. Jackie
had purchased it from a white education professor at Fort Valley
State College before the professor left the college and moved away.

The goldish-yellow wood frame house had a screened front porch.
I loved it because it reminded me of my Aunt Gladys and Uncle
Hutch's house in Ohio. I also loved screened front porches because
of the one on my grandparents' lake house in northern Minnesota.

Herman wanted to start an herb farm here. The house sat on an
embankment above the country road, and we could sit on the porch
and look off across the fields on the other side.

We bought the house in 1978, but before we got our furniture moved in all the way, someone shot through the house with a high-powered rifle. We later found out which relative of our closer neighbors had done that, but not because of any diligence of the sheriff's department in Macon County.

I cried for a minute when we saw it, but we went ahead and moved in. I figured it had to be a coward who came and did his dirty work when no one was home.

Alex was born in 1979, and we developed friendly relations with most of our nearby neighbors. They included white and black farmers, although the farming on the half-sand, half-clay, land out there was not large scale or highly profitable.

In December 1992, we moved back to Peach County, to a house we had built on property we bought from Herman's grandmother's cousin, Mrs. Leola Arnold. It was less than a mile from Stallworth Trailer Park, and on the same road, a now paved Old Marshallville Road that became part of State University Drive, which once was South Macon Street, on the black side of town. I recently noticed a white family living on State University Drive out our way.

As Buddy Smisson once said, "It's coming."

Respects to those who have died:

Many family members, students, colleagues, and townspeople included in this memoir have passed away. I wish they were here to read and reminisce. I cherish my memories of them.

Acknowledgements

I would like to acknowledge the impact that all those named in this memoir have had on my life, and especially my husband Herman and our sons Aaron and Alex. I thank Herman for his support during the years I have worked on the book and Aaron and Alex for cheering me on. The Parsons, our Georgia family, have kept me connected to the culture I first became a part of in the late sixties when I came to Fort Valley. I am grateful for these life experiences. Thanks also to my brother Peter Wallace for his input on the manuscript. I am especially grateful to my parents, Irving and Lovella Wallace, for instilling in me the belief that we should respect all people and treat everyone as equals.

I'd like to thank Margaret H. Rodeheaver as well as Chad R. Allen and my fellow BookCamp members for the help they provided with revising, editing, and preparing to publish and launch the book. Wilmetta Langston, Fort Valley State College Class of 1958, provided invaluable help locating information and photographs in the FVSU Heritage Room, especially the photograph of the neon sign over the entrance that I saw when I arrived in 1968 and the photo of me with other new faculty members that fall.

About the author

ANNA R. HOLLOWAY, PHD, is a retired Professor of English, writer, and editor. She is originally from the Midwest and now in the South, and she and her husband have two sons. During her forty-six years at the black institution, Fort Valley State University, Anna taught writing, literature, journalism, technical writing, and editing and served many years as advisor to the student creative writing magazine. She retired as Dean of Graduate Studies and Extended Education. In addition to family, friends, and cats, she cares deeply about bringing about understanding among people of different backgrounds and opinions.

AnnaHollowayWrites.com

Made in United States
Troutdale, OR
05/11/2024

19804873R20146